I0783167

**Imprint**

Ines and Frank Lohrmann

# Old home remedies
# for ailments and well-being

An extensive collection of old home remedies from Europe

**Over 2000 tips and more than 500 recipes**

First edition 2024


**Publisher**
ODIN Verlagsservice
Siegener Strasse 2
D-51545 Waldbroel
Germany

kind be accepted for any disadvantages or damages resulting from the hints, applications, and procedures described in the book.

# TABLE OF CONTENT

# TABLE OF CONTENT

# TABLE OF CONTENT

# TABLE OF CONTENT

## RECIPES

## PREFACE

Home remedies are remedies that provide assistance with minor problems using household means. Home remedies are often historically transmitted and often contain the knowledge that has been accumulated over generations, transmitted in writing, sometimes only orally. Based on observations of the environment, sometimes only on assumptions, home remedies can have an effect, but they may not.

In this book, we aim to provide a list of home remedies that have been used in the past and are often still used today. However, we do not make any statements about their effectiveness or ineffectiveness.

Under no circumstances should home remedies be used to replace medical advice - often only a trained pharmacist or a doctor can make the correct diagnosis. Home remedies should not encourage careless self-diagnosis and self-medication.

Many minor complaints may also have their cause in serious illnesses - under no circumstances should a doctor's visit be postponed or replaced, as the time factor is also crucial for healing.

In this book, we only provide an overview of which home remedies have historically been used for various minor ailments or complaints. We do not encourage you to treat your illnesses or complaints with home remedies. Our list of old home remedies may also contain incorrect, incomplete, or misleading information. Please critically evaluate each piece of information with other sources. We do not accept liability for damages arising from the application of information provided here.

The information provided is based on evaluated literature, personal and known uses, as well as hearsay - the information provided may also be incorrect, outdated, or obsolete.

We have excluded mystical, ritualistic, and religious home remedies, as well as those based on animal products. Therefore, you will not find remedies here that involve cremated frogs or crow's blood, nor rituals for exorcism or healing prayers.

Much of the information is based on folklore sources, which may have incorporated false or incorrect experiences. We do not provide treatment advice here, but only list old knowledge, which may also be completely false, incorrect, or misleading.

If you have health complaints, always consult your doctor or pharmacist and trust them as necessary.

## HISTORICAL BACKGROUND

Since the existence of humans, they have had to deal with parasites, injuries, and diseases. The first medicine used was home remedies, based on personal and others' observations of the body within the context of the surrounding environment in nature and the household.

Often, these observations, as well as in the history of medicine, were associated with divine or pagan religious practices. In all ancient cultures, one can find the connection between faith, rituals, home remedies, and hope for healing. Gods were considered both the cause of diseases and healers in times of need. In ancient China, this gave rise to Traditional Chinese Medicine (TCM), while in India, it led to the principles of Ayurveda (The Science of Life). The modern European medicine evolved from medical approaches established in ancient Greece at least 3,000 years ago. The beginnings of Greek and Egyptian medicine also assumed that health and illness were subject to divine influences. From this arose distinct castes, whose main task was healing. They acted as intermediaries between the gods and the sick, initially the shamans, and in later cultures, the priest-physicians. Ritual acts ensured mental and physical health. Oracles were consulted, and miraculous healings were recorded for posterity.

After the collapse of the Roman Empire, medicine fell into the hands of monks and clergy who dealt with wound healing. In 1162, the clergy were forbidden to engage in bloody medicine with the declaration "Ecclesia abhorret a sanguine" (The Church abhors blood), leading to other professional groups taking over large parts of medicine. Thus, barbers took on the medically significant "bloodletting" practice. Barbers and wound doctors were employed as field surgeons in military service during wartime conflicts, where they performed medical and surgical tasks. Quacks, bathers, barbers, lithotomists, and wound doctors traveled as itinerant people from market town to market town, offering their services, sometimes to the benefit, sometimes to the detriment, of the sick or those seeking healing. Qualifications were not necessarily required, so many charlatans, rogues, and fraudsters were among this traveling population.

Under these circumstances, it is not surprising that the population often preferred to stick to tried and tested methods and procedures rather than entrusting themselves to the risky hands of the physicians of the time. When caution, prayer, and amulets failed, and one was afflicted by ailments, illness, and suffering, people preferred to make their own medicine based on old knowledge, often derived from actual experiences, or followed instructions promising healing or relief. If the affliction persisted, one could still turn to the hands of the healers of the time or seek improvement from the knowledge of wise women or village witches, who were both revered and often outcasts of society, as they were also accused of cursing with their knowledge or causing disease, hardship, death of livestock, and worse. When these wise individuals were called upon, they used their knowledge of nature and human physiology, accumulated over generations, sometimes adding magic and a small spell to ensure that the suffering improved. If that didn't work, it was usually considered God's will; if it did succeed in dispelling the suffering, the wise woman or healer had surely gained a new client. Sometimes, a simple home remedy or simply time, which the affliction needed to improve, was enough.

Even today, wise women in rural areas perform religious or pagan rituals, incantations, and healing prayers, which often lead to improvement. One reason for the improvement through incantation is surely to be seen in psychology because those who believe in the effectiveness will be surprised by the effectiveness. The same certainly applies nowadays to many products and treatment methods such as homeopathy, Schuessler salts, or Bach flower therapy, which often assume mechanisms of action that contradict normal science or concentrations of active ingredients where there is no active ingredient present, or the concentration of any impurity exceeds the concentration of the active ingredient. In experiments and studies, pure placebos have also proven their effectiveness.

We aim to focus here on old and well-known experience-based home remedies, excluding those based on animal products, rituals, mystical glorifications, pagan and religious rituals, prayers, and incantations.

Home remedies, in this sense, are not only self-made remedies for rubbing on or ingesting but also simple methods to provide relief for discomfort and minor ailments. This can consist of behavioral guidelines for prevention and relief, as well as procedures such as compresses, especially chest compresses, neck compresses, or calf compresses, but also baths such as steam baths, foot baths, and poultices or plasters.

A large area is occupied by herbal substances, the effects of which have been observed, recorded, or passed down orally from generation to generation, especially since the Middle Ages

## COLLECTED HOME REMEDIES

The following contributions contain only general information and should not be used as self-diagnosis or self-treatment. All information provided here is intended solely for general knowledge and should not replace a visit to a doctor, as only a trained physician can provide diagnoses and treatment recommendations.

### 1. FATIGUE, EXHAUSTION

One of the simplest remedies was and still is: simply drinking a glass of hot water. An alternative that brings fresh energy is also 1 glass of apple juice, mixed with 1 tablespoon of honey. For fatigue, foot baths can help. Sugar creates new energy. When in a hurry, sugar-rich fruits like bananas or apples will do. A foot bath of 20 minutes with 1 tablespoon of savory or 3 tablespoons of comfrey can be helpful. Comfrey is especially recommended for physical fatigue. Alternating baths or showers with warm and cold water are also helpful; this effect can be enhanced by vigorously brushing the feet. One should end with the cold bath or shower. To strengthen general well-being, especially in spring, a nettle cure with nettle tea is recommended. Drink 2 cups of nettle tea per day for three weeks. Liquor and schnapps were also commonly made from the plant. To prevent exhaustion and during heavy work, especially at high altitudes, it was common in the mountains to drink a tea made from Alpine mugwort (Artemisia umbelliformis) or to chew the herb. A course of apple cider vinegar and honey should revive the spirits.

APPLE CIDER VINEGAR REGIMEN

> Mix 3 tablespoons of apple cider vinegar in a glass of water
> with 1 tablespoon of honey and drink daily in the morning
> for several weeks.

Lavender was a remedy commonly used as a household remedy.

Lavender sugar should be consumed by eating 1 teaspoon of it when experiencing early signs of exhaustion.

## LAVENDER SUGAR

> Lavender sugar is prepared by mixing 10 tablespoons of
> sugar with 2 tablespoons of lavender flowers and storing
> them in a sealed jar. After 10 days, it is ready to use.

## NETTLE TEA

> Pour 1-2 teaspoons of finely chopped nettle leaves into a
> cup of boiling water, and let it steep for 5 minutes before
> straining and drinking.

To prevent it, it is recommended to spend time outdoors frequently. Additionally, a balanced and vitamin-rich diet can support this. For breakfast, you can drink mixtures of apple juice, carrot juice, orange juice, and lemon juice.

As a preventive measure, it is recommended to undergo a tea cure in the spring.

## SPRING TEA CURE

> 2 tbsp birch leaves
> 2 tbsp raspberry leaves
> 2 tbsp wild strawberry leaves
> 2 tbsp black currant leaves
> Infuse each with 1 cup of boiling water, let steep for 5
> minutes, and drink 2-3 times a day without sweetening.

Fir shoot tea was used against fatigue and spring fatigue.

## SPRUCE SHOOT TEA

> One adds 1 teaspoon of fresh spruce shoot tips to a cup
> and pours boiling water over them. Let it steep covered for
> 10 minutes, then strain. The tea can also be sweetened
> with some honey.

An elecampane wine was also recommended for weakness. This
was said to be particularly helpful for emaciation, decline,
exhaustion, and general weakness.

## ELECAMPANE WINE

> 4 tablespoons of grated elecampane root are steeped in 1
> liter of white wine. The glass is sealed and left to stand
> warm for 3 weeks. Then, the liquid is filtered, and the root
> is squeezed out. Before the main meal, a shot glass full of
> the liquid is taken.

## 2.   ABSCESS, ULCERS, INFLAMMATIONS

Poultices made from bread, milk, and saffron were used to accelerate maturation in purulent inflammations. A similar effect is believed to be achieved by binding a roasted and cut onion overnight with a bandage over the center of the inflammation.

Applying fresh, crushed chamomile herb is very helpful for ulcers.

Placing the white inner skin of eggs on the abscess is said to alleviate suffering. It is also believed to help with suppurations of the nail bed when applied.

Similarly, placing warm scrambled eggs on the abscess is believed to yield the same results.

A very old remedy is to apply a honey compress to the abscess. Honey can also be mixed with crushed burdock root to enhance its effectiveness. This compress should be renewed several times a day.

If ulcers refused to heal or were suppurating, ground larch bark was sprinkled on them.

Foresters and farmers have used rubbing with spruce resin ointment or fir resin ointment to alleviate symptoms.

SPRUCE RESIN OINTMENT OR FIR RESIN OINTMENT

> Heat 1/2 butter and 1/2 beef tallow gently, mix 3 tbsp honey, some pine resin or spruce resin, and a few drops of linseed oil to form an ointment.

Apply a poultice of oatmeal to inflamed joints, wash off thoroughly in the morning.

## OATMEAL POULTICE

> Heat oatmeal flour or oat flakes in a small amount of water or milk, mix it with lanolin, and apply the paste to a cloth or bandage. Wrap the joint with it overnight.

Using poultices made from bean flour was also common, especially to help mature purulent ulcers that refuse to burst.

Rinsing with chamomile tea.

## CHAMOMILE TEA

> Pour boiling water over 1-2 teaspoons of chamomile and let it steep for 5 minutes.

Apply calendula ointment to the inflammation.

## CALENDULA OINTMENT

> 100 g clarified butter
> 4 tbsp oil or olive oil
> 30 g marigold flowers
> Heat the clarified butter with the oil. Then add the

marigold flowers. Keep it hot for 30 minutes, but do not boil. Remove from the heat, cover, and let it stand for a day. Heat again, strain through a sieve, squeezing out the flowers. Now add 30 g beeswax to the oil and let it melt. Mix everything well and fill into small jars.

Apply a compress with cabbage leaves to the inflamed area.

## COMPRESS WITH CABBAGE LEAVES

Remove the tough rib from a cabbage leaf, then roll it flat with a rolling pin. Apply the leaf overnight and secure it with a bandage or a linen cloth.

Wraps with hot birch leaves are also said to be helpful.

## BIRCH LEAF WRAPS

One places birch leaves in hot water and then makes wraps out of the hot birch leaves by wrapping them in cloths and applying them. After some time, the wraps are renewed.

# 3.  ALLERGY, HAY FEVER

All information and home remedies provided are for informational purposes only. They do not represent current scientific knowledge and are not intended for self-medication. Diagnosis and medication can only be carried out by a doctor or pharmacist.

To combat hay fever, the white inner skin of lemons and oranges, boiled in water for 10 minutes and sweetened with a little honey, is said to help. Take 1 teaspoon of this mixture in the morning, afternoon, and evening.

Drinking nettle tea over several weeks is also believed to alleviate hay fever symptoms.

An old remedy is nasal irrigation with water.

Additionally, drinking eyebright tea has been recommended for hay fever relief.

## 4.  FEAR, ANXIETY DISORDERS

An old remedy for anxiety is to eat chocolate. Chocolate with high cocoa content is believed to be more effective in this regard.

Another old remedy for anxiety is to place dried herbs such as hops, thyme, rosemary, and valerian in a small cloth bag and place it next to the pillow overnight.

Also, a relaxation tea can help.

### RELAXIATION TEA

- 20 g Valerian root
- 10 g Hop flower
- 10 g Peppermint leaves
- 10 g Lemon balm leaves

- 5 g Orange peel

Mix all ingredients well. Pour 3 teaspoons of this mixture into a cup of boiling water, let it steep for 10 minutes, then strain.

Chewed calamus root is also said to help with anxiety and have a calming effect.

Plenty of exercise and outdoor activities can dispel anxiety.

Other well-known remedies for anxiety include valerian tea, hops tea, lemon balm tea, and St. John's Wort as a tincture or tea.

## 5. APHTHAE

Rinse the mouth frequently with cold water and drink cold water.

Apply a mixture of honey and turmeric to the affected areas.

### HONEY-TURMERIC MIXTURE

1 tablespoon honey
1 teaspoon turmeric

Mix well.

Avoiding hot or spicy foods, consuming cold foods and drinks, and eating ice can be helpful.

Applying radish juice, papaya juice, or aloe vera to the aphthous ulcer can be very beneficial.

Avoiding pork.

Avoiding stress.

Rinsing with chamomile tea, sage tea, lemon balm tea, or green tea, or applying the corresponding tinctures to the aphthous ulcer, is also helpful.

Applying lemon juice or baking soda is also said to have a positive effect.

## SAGE TEA

1-2 teaspoons of dried sage
infuse with 1 cup of boiling water, let steep for 5 minutes.

## LEMON BALM TEA

1-2 teaspoons of dried lemon balm
infuse with 1 cup of boiling water, let steep for 5 minutes.

Apply aloe vera extract or gel to the Aphthae.

## 6.  LOSS OF APPETITE

Yarrow tea with a bit of caraway before meals can increase appetite.

Chewing dried juniper berries between meals may help stimulate appetite.

Eating a few chewed caraway seeds or having a salad before meals can also boost appetite.

Certain spices are believed to naturally stimulate appetite, such as caraway, ginger, and cinnamon.

Taking a teaspoon of mustard before meals is said to stimulate appetite. Other common remedies include sour pickles or gentian schnapps.

Wormwood tea before meals can also increase appetite, as well as getting plenty of exercise outdoors.

### WORMWOOD TEA

1 teaspoon of wormwood herb
steeped in a cup of boiling water for 10 minutes, covered, then strained.

Drinking lavender flower tea before meals is also said to stimulate the appetite.

## LAVENDER FLOWER TEA

> Pour 2 teaspoons of lavender flowers into 1 cup of boiling water, let steep for 10 minutes, and strain.

Appetite stimulant tea was a popular home remedy, especially in the southern German-speaking regions.

## APPETITE-STIMULATING TEA

> - 15 g bitter clover
> - 15 g wormwood herb
> - 15 g juniper berries
>
> Boil in 1 liter of water and reduce to 500 ml. Strain and take 1-2 tablespoons before meals.

Other teas that were said to have an appetite-stimulating effect included hop tea, tea made from centaury, rose hips, coriander, cinnamon bark, or chamomile.

Alant is also said to boost appetite. For this, a small piece of the alant root is chewed, or alant tincture is used. With the tincture, you can take up to 20 drops up to 3 times a day.

## ALECAMPANE TINCTURE

> One fills a glass halfway with crushed alant root. Then, one
> fills the glass with brandy or grain alcohol and lets it steep
> for 5 weeks in a closed container at a warm place. The
> liquid is strained, the remaining root is squeezed, and then
> the liquid is filled into dark bottles.

## 7.  ARTERIOSCLEROSIS, STROKE

Preventively, one can consume plenty of fruits and sauerkraut and engage in regular outdoor activities.

It's advisable to avoid lard and pork.

Mistletoe tea was a remedy for a weak heart, stroke, and arteriosclerosis.

An ant steam bath was believed to help alleviate trembling limbs in the case of a stroke.

## MISTLETOE TEA

> 1 teaspoon of mistletoe herb is poured over with a cup of
> cold water. Let the cup stand covered overnight and strain
> the next day. The liquid can now be drunk cold or warm in
> small sips.

> It's important to only steep mistletoe herb with cold water,
> as many toxins of the mistletoe would be dissolved inhot
> water

From the 19th century onwards, hawthorn tea was used to strengthen the heart. One cup should be consumed in the morning and one in the evening. Hawthorn tincture was taken up to 3 times a day, with 15 drops each time. Hawthorn is also believed to help with low blood pressure.

## HAWTHORN TEA

> 2 teaspoons of dried or fresh flowers or leaves are infused with 1 cup of boiling water. Let it steep covered for 20 minutes, then strain. The tea can also be sweetened with a little honey.

## HAWTHORN TINCTURE

> A glass is filled halfway with fresh hawthorn leaves and flowers, pressed down, and covered with brandy (or vodka). Then place it in a warm spot and shake it daily. After about 4 weeks, strain and press the herb well. Pour the liquid into dark bottles and seal them.

Garlic, leeks, and onions are the vegetables believed to have good effects on the blood and heart strengthening. It was recommended to eat plenty of them.

If the smell bothers, a glass of garlic milk was consumed daily.

## GARLIC MILK

> Crush 2 garlic cloves and simmer them with a glass of milk for 5 minutes. The milk should be consumed warm.

## 8.  ARTHRITIS, OSTEOARTHRITIS

A bee resin ointment was supposed to help with arthritis. Bee resin is the substance with which bees seal their hive entrance to the necessary size. Today, it is known as propolis. To make an ointment, the bee resin was mixed with honey, beeswax, and oil.

Rosehip tea was also supposed to provide relief and prevention.

## ROSEHIP TEA

> 1-2 teaspoons of deseeded rose hips are poured over with a cup of boiling water and left to steep for 10 minutes.

Millet is believed to have preventive effects. One can drink the cooking water or apply millet as a poultice.

Celery water was also commonly consumed to positively influence inflammation.

## CELERY WATER

> Chop celery and boil it in water. Then strain it. Drink one
> cup of the liquid three times a day.

Baths in saltwater are believed to have a positive effect.

Applying orange peels with the white side on the joints is believed to alleviate pain.

Wraps with cabbage leaves are also thought to help with pain.

## CABBAGE LEAF COMPRESS

> The tough midrib is cut from cabbage leaves. Then, the
> cabbage leaf is rolled with a rolling pin or a bottle until
> cabbage juice is released. Now, place the leaves on the
> affected areas and wrap them with a linen cloth. Leave it
> on for several hours.

Quark compresses are said to alleviate joint pain.

## QUARK COMPRESS

> Mix 250 g of quark with 1 tablespoon of olive oil
> thoroughly and refrigerate the quark before use. Then
> apply it to the joints, wrap with a linen cloth, and let it sit
> for about 30 minutes. Afterwards, wash it off with water.

## 9.  ASTHMA, SHORTNESS OF BREATH, BREATHLESSNESS

A steam bath with chamomile tea alleviates shortness of breath and asthma.

Drinking anise tea is a home remedy for asthma and shortness of breath.

### ANISE TEA

1 teaspoon of anise seeds Crush the seeds and pour them into 1 cup of boiling water. Let it steep for 10 minutes, then strain.

One should drink one cup of asthma tea in the morning and two cups in the evening.

### ASTHMA TEA

> 50 g goosegrass
> 50 g St. John's wort
> 30 g orange blossoms
> 20 g lavender blossoms
> Infuse 1 teaspoon of the mixture with boiling water, let it steep for 5 minutes, and drink.

One can take a few tablespoons of freshly pressed radish juice in the morning, or eat a tablespoon of grated horseradish with honey in the morning, noon, and evening.

Grated horseradish mixed with water, taken as a tablespoon in the evening, is said to prevent nighttime attacks.

Freshly grated horseradish, placed on the inner surfaces of the forearms, is believed to prevent attacks.

Consuming crushed yellow mustard in bread, meat broth, or tea in the morning and evening is also said to clear the chest.

A decoction of the marsh snake's head (Polygala amarella) root is also believed to be helpful against asthma and shortness of breath.

## SWAMP CROSSFLOWER TEA

> Boil 1 tablespoon of swamp crossflower root with 500 ml of water for 15 minutes. This amount corresponds to approximately 3 cups of tea, drunk throughout the day.

The cooking broth or water from vegetable asparagus was a home remedy for shortness of breath.

Beech bark tea is a home remedy for shortness of breath.

## BEECH BARK TEA

> 1 teaspoon of beech bark in a cup, pour boiling water over it, let it steep covered for 10 minutes, then strain.

The decoction of boiled garlic is said to help with shortness of breath.

Speedwell tea is said to be beneficial for asthma.

## SPEEDWELL TEA

> 1 teaspoon of dried speedwell herb (Veronica officinalis) is infused with 1 cup of boiling water, covered, allowed to steep for 5 minutes, and then strained.

During an attack, soaking the hands in hot water can be helpful. Avoid using feather beds. Applying cold compresses to the chest can alleviate the attack.

Avoiding poor air quality and exposure to fumes from paint, varnish, and cleaning products is essential.

Engaging in plenty of outdoor activities in the woods and fresh air reduces the susceptibility to asthma attacks.

Inhaling the scent of crushed pine or fir needles is said to help with asthma.

Foresters have chewed pine resin for asthma or shortness of breath.

Applying compresses with horseradish, onion, and honey should also be helpful.

## HORSERADISH-ONION-HONEY COMPRESSES

> 3 tablespoons of grated horseradish are mixed with 1 tablespoon of honey and 1 tablespoon of finely chopped onion. Then apply it to the chest and cover with a linen cloth, leaving it on for approximately 15-20 minutes.

During cold and damp weather, it's advisable to protect the mouth with a cloth or scarf, inhale through the nose, and exhale through the mouth.

Tea made from Mexican Tea (Dysphania ambrosioides) was also a remedy for asthma, as well as for lung ailments and shortness of breath.

Additionally, teas made from mullein, goosefoot, St. John's wort, lavender, mint, and lemon balm are good home remedies for breathlessness or asthma.

## 10. BAD BREATH

To combat bad breath, rinsing the mouth and brushing teeth are helpful.

Mouthwashes with saltwater also aid in fighting bad breath. For this, one teaspoon of salt per glass of water is used. However, it's important to ensure that the salt doesn't contain additives like iodine, anti-caking agents, etc.

Gargling with black tea is also effective as it has antibacterial properties that prevent bad breath. If bad breath is caused by consuming garlic, chewing herbs like peppermint, sage, and parsley can help. Drinking milk or consuming cottage cheese can also alleviate the odor.

Elderflower tea and chamomile tea are suitable for gargling to combat bad breath.

Chewing a clove, fennel seeds, cardamom, dill seeds, anise seeds, caraway seeds, horseradish, a juniper berry, or a coffee bean, or sucking on eucalyptus lozenges are also effective methods.

Gargling with mouthwash, saltwater, or diluted vinegar water was also a common practice.

## ALUM GARGLE

4 g alum

100 ml water

Dissolve the alum in the water.

## 11. BELCHING, HICCUPS

To stop hiccups, there are many home remedies. Holding your breath for as long as possible is said to be effective. Slowly drinking water while holding your breath may also help. Controlled and regular breathing can also help get rid of hiccups. Additionally, sucking on a stone or an ice cube is believed to help stop hiccups.

To stop belching, a sweet, peeled almond was chewed and eaten.

Chamomile tea, fennel tea, anise tea, ginger tea, or caraway tea are also remedies of choice for persistent belching.

## 12. EYE, REMOVING INSECTS OR FOREIGN BODIES FROM

One rolls a small piece of paper together, moistens the tip, and removes the foreign object with it.

Gently wash the eye with water.

Smell freshly cut onions and hold them under the eye. The tears might flush out the foreign object.

## 13. BURST CAPILLARIES IN GEHE EYE

Place raw, still warm veal meat on the eye.

Here, a compress with fennel tea could also help.

## 14. EYES, TIREDOR EXHAUSTED

The still warm pulp of a baked apple is said to help with redness when applied to closed eyes for about 10 minutes, then washed off.

Short outings in nature support the eyes and relax them.

Consciously closing the eyes for 5 minutes relaxes both the eyes and the mind.

Slices of green cucumber placed on the eyes for 10 minutes relax them, providing freshness and reducing dark circles.

## 15. EYE PROBLEMS, VISION PROBLEMS

Binding some celandine on the eyes overnight.

Also, an eyebright wine was very often used. In Italy and France, eyebright was probably used even more intensively than in Germany. One drinks about 50 ml or a liqueur glass full of eyebright wine daily.

EYEBRIGHT WINE

- • 2 handfuls of eyebright herb
- • 750 ml white wine

Put the herb in a sealable jar and pour the white wine over it. Now let it sit in a warm, non-sunny place for 14 days, shaking it daily. Then strain the liquid.

In other recipes, eyebright was fermented together with the grapes.

When experiencing vision problems, eyes were often treated with compresses soaked in anise tea. A piece of cloth was soaked in anise tea and placed on the eyes. Washing the eyes with anise tea was also common.

Wormwood juice made from fresh wormwood, mixed with honey and applied as a compress on the eye, is said to not only help weak eyes but also combat eye inflammations. Compresses with rosemary tea, wormwood tea, or hyssop tea can also be used.

The following herbal mixture, added to meals daily in a teaspoonful, is said to strengthen the eyesight.

## EYE HERBS

2 tablespoons of dill seeds
2 tablespoons of peppercorns
2 tablespoons of cinnamon
2 tablespoons of fennel seeds
4 EL Fenchelsamen

> From the mixture add 1 teaspoon to the food.

## 16. EYE INFLAMMATION, CONCONDICTIVITY

Particularly drafts can lead to conjunctivitis, which is why they should be avoided.

A compress with boiled chamomile tea or black tea, where the tea is wrapped in a cloth and placed on the eyes, is a helpful home remedy for an eye inflammation.

One can rinse glued eyes with lukewarm water.

Applying a quince seed compress was an old home remedy.

### QUINCE SEED COMPRESS

> Shake 10 quince seeds vigorously in 100 ml of water for at least 5 minutes, then strain through a cloth. Dip a cloth into the liquid and apply it as a compress to the eye.

Dab the eye with eyebright tea. You can also drink the tea to support from the inside. An eyebright compress is also helpful.

### EYEBRIGHT TEA

> - 1 teaspoon dried eyebright herb or

> • 2 teaspoon fresh eyebright herb
>
> Pour over with one cup of boiling water, let it steep covered for 10 minutes.

For conjunctivitis, you can rinse the eye with eyebright tea to which you add a little salt. It is important to filter the tea well for this purpose. A compress with rose petals should also be helpful.

## ROSE PETAL COMPRESS

> A handful of rose petals are poured over with a handful of boiling water. Let it steep covered for 5 minutes, then strain. Now dip a cloth into it and place it on the eyes.

Using sage compresses, applied three times a day, should also help with inflamed eyes.

## SAGE COMPRESS

> 2 teaspoons of sage leaves are steeped in 1 cup of boiling water, covered, for 5 minutes, then strained. Wait until the liquid reaches body temperature. Now, soak linen cloths in it and place them on the closed eyes.

If the eyes are stuck together, a compress with walnut decoction should help loosen the adhesions.

## WALNUT COMPRESS

1 walnut leaf, thoroughly washed, is simmered in 500 ml of water for 10 minutes and strained. Soak a cloth in the decoction and place it on the closed eyes for about 10 minutes.

A rinse with turmeric or compresses with marigold or sage should also help.

## TURMERIC RINSE

1 teaspoon of ground turmeric, steeped in a cup of boiling water. Let it sit covered for 15 minutes, then strain. Filter the liquid well through paper (coffee filter, kitchen paper) or cloth. The eye is rinsed with the warmed liquid 3 times a day. You can also add a little salt.

## MARIGOLD COMPRESS

2 teaspoons of marigold in 2 cups of water, bring to a boil and let it steep covered for 15 minutes. Now immerse a linen cloth in the warm liquid and place it on the eye. This procedure should be repeated several times throughout the day.

## SAGE COMPRESSES

> Bring 2 teaspoons of marigold flowers to a boil in 2 cups of
> water, then let it simmer covered for 15 minutes. Next,
> soak a linen cloth in the warm liquid and place it on the
> eye. Repeat this procedure several times throughout the
> day.

A compress with oak bark tea should also help with eye inflammation. Dip a cloth in the oak bark tea and place it on the eyes. Repeat several times a day.

## OAK BARK TEA

> 1 teaspoon of chopped oak bark, boiled in two cups of
> water for three minutes, then strained and allowed to cool
> covered.

When eyes were sore and stuck together, it was recommended to boil a dried poppy seed head in milk, dip a cloth in it, and apply it as a compress to the eyes.

In Russia, a compress with linden bark was used for eye inflammations.

## LINDEN BARK POULTICE

> One scrapes the bark, including the inner white part, from
> a fresh branch of the linden tree. This is then poured over
> with 250 ml of cold water. Afterwards, the bark is beaten
> with a mallet and then dipped back into the water until

> mucus forms. This mucus is placed on a linen cloth, which
> is then folded and applied to the eyes.

## 17. EYE BAGS

Among the Romans, a mixture of honey and roasted garlic applied as a salve was a remedy for combating dark circles under the eyes.

A more modern approach is a compress made with black tea steeped in boiling water and wrapped in a cloth.

Slices of fresh green cucumber placed on the eyes are said to relax the eyes and reduce dark circles.

Cold compresses, such as ice wrapped in a cloth, can also help. Some people also hold a cold spoon against the dark circles.

You can also apply a quark mask.

### CURD MASK

> 200 g curd is mixed with 1 teaspoon of olive oil and 2 teaspoons
> of lemon juice. This mask is applied to the dark circles under
> the eyes and left on for approximately 1-2 hours.

## 18. WATERY EYES

15 drops of eyebright tincture in a glass of water to wash and moisten the eyes more frequently.

## 19. FACIAL RASH

Boil tea from buckthorn bark and shepherd's purse, mix it with some cooking oil, and apply it to the affected areas.

### TEA FROM BUCKTHORN BARK AND SHEPHERD'S PURSE

1 teaspoon of buckthorn bark
1 teaspoon of shepherd's purse
Boil in water for 2 minutes and strain.

The skin was often washed with strong soapy water to improve rashes.

## 20. RASH, ECZEMA

Washes with mistletoe tea and compresses with mistletoe herb were a remedy in folk medicine for eczema and rash.

Among the Romans, a ointment made from garlic, a little salt, and olive oil was a remedy for skin rash.

## 21. EMACIATION, LOSS OF STRENGTH, CONSUMPTION

Eating honey and drinking milk. Drinking chicken broth for breakfast.

To rebuild emaciated individuals, sweet beer soups were also commonly used.

These were prepared with egg, honey or sugar, and also flour.

Mixing 8 tablespoons of goat butter with 4 tablespoons of honey, taking 1 tablespoon of it in the morning and evening, is said to be invigorating.

Blackberry tea, sweetened with rock candy, is said to have a positive effect on the lungs.

Tea made from speedwell and sage tea are good remedies to help with chest problems.

Snail broth was once a proven remedy in folk medicine for emaciation.

## SNAIL BROTH

6-8 large snails were pulled out of the crushed shell with a fork, cleaned of their gall, rubbed with salt, briefly fried in fat, and boiled with 500 ml of water. A cup of the broth was drunk in the morning. The snail broth can also be made more effective by adding grated deer horn and cooked pearl barley.

Drinking up to 500 ml of freshly grated and squeezed cucumber juice daily is said to have positive effects.

## 22. SWOLLEN LEGS

For a long time, a common home remedy for swollen legs was to rub them with rubbing alcohol in the evening.

Support stockings were common, especially for prolonged standing.

Foot baths with comfrey or rosemary were popular for swollen legs. Alternating cold/warm foot baths were also used.

Another remedy was to elevate the legs to support blood flow. Sleeping with elevated feet was also believed to be helpful.

## 23. RESTLESS LEGS

What is commonly known as restless legs syndrome, or "Restless Leg" in modern terms, was also a problem people struggled with in the past. When going to bed, the legs would twitch, making it difficult to fall asleep...

One remedy was to take a 10-minute walk before bedtime.

A cold foot bath before going to bed was also believed to help.

Others recommended foot baths with a addition of crushed mustard seeds briefly boiled in water.

The seeds of the cowhage plant - Mucuna pruriens - were also recommended, for example, as a tea made from about 1 gram of seeds. However, the bean is toxic, and experimentation should be avoided!

## 24. SPIDER VEINS

Alternating cold and warm baths on the legs were believed to help.

Compresses made from green tea and black tea were also thought to be helpful.

## 25. FLATULENCE

Bloating is also determined by diet. If you experience particularly strong bloating after certain foods, you can avoid them to reduce symptoms. Foods that are particularly "bloating-intensive" include cabbage, beans, peas, fatty meats, very fresh bread, etc.

Eating behavior can also contribute to bloating. Talking a lot while eating can cause you to swallow a lot of air, which needs to be expelled later.

If you experience bloating, applying heat to the stomach can help. Grain pillows, cherry stone pillows, or a hot water bottle on the abdomen can provide relief.

Extracts and tinctures of wormwood, gentian, and milk thistle are also good remedies for fighting bloating.

Caraway, anise, peppermint, and fennel were effective remedies for bloating and stomach problems. You can chew and swallow a pinch of these seeds or drink their tea individually or mixed. Avoid adding sweeteners.

## ANTI-FLATULENCE TEA

- 3 tablespoons caraway seeds
- 3 tablespoons  anise seeds
- 3 tablespoons fennel seeds

Mix them together well. Take 1 teaspoon of this mixture and boil it in a pot. Let it steep for 10 minutes, then strain and drink.

Also, chamomile tea was also consumed to alleviate flatulence.

## 26. CYSTITIS

Here are some old tips:

Preventatively, always empty your bladder completely.

After intercourse, go to the toilet and empty your bladder.

At the first signs of symptoms, take a warm bath and drink plenty of fluids. Keep the lower body warm, and a hot water bottle between the legs can also help.

Diet can also contribute to urinary tract health. Avoid meat and opt for rice, grain porridge, and vegetables. Too much coffee and alcohol can be counterproductive.

Infusions of watercress or daisies are believed to have a favorable effect on urinary tract infections. To prepare, boil 2-3 teaspoons of the herbs in a pot with a large cup of water, let it steep covered for 10 minutes, then strain.

Rosehip tea is also a home remedy.

Dandelion tea could also be helpful.

Sitz baths with chamomile are said to be very effective.

## DANDELION TEA

- 1 teaspoon dried dandelion leaves
- 1 teaspoon dried dandelion roots

Place them in a pot, pour 1 cup of water over them, bring to a brief boil, then let it steep covered for 15 minutes. Finally, strain the mixture.

An old remedy is also bearberry leaf tea.

## BEARBERRY LEAVES TEA

1 heaping teaspoon of bearberry leaves is poured over with 1 cup of cold water. The tea stands covered for about 10 hours and is then strained. It is important to prepare the

tea with cold water and to use it only up to 3 times a day for 1 week.

For urinary tract infections, diuretic teas such as tea made from horsetail, goldenrod, and nettle can help.

Birch leaf tea, drunk on an empty stomach, should also help.

## BIRCH LEAF TEA

2 teaspoons of crushed birch leaves pour over with 1 cup of boiling water, let it steep for 15 minutes, and strain.

Eating grated horseradish or watercress should also help with urinary tract infections.

An old remedy is also a sitz bath or steam bath with chamomile for the lower area.

.

## CHAMOMILE STEAM BATH „BOTTOM"

3 teaspoons of chamomile are placed in an old pot and boiled with 300 ml of water. The pot is then placed in the toilet bowl, and the person sits on the toilet. The lower body and the toilet are wrapped well with a blanket.

As a preventive measure, one can also eat radishes, garlic, cucumber seeds, or pumpkin seeds. Snacking on pumpkin seeds also has a good and strengthening effect on the bladder.

Watercress, primroses, nettles, and elderberries are said to positively influence kidney inflammation and kidney pelvis inflammation.

Warm baths, especially at the beginning, were also recommended.

A bladder tea from the realm of folk medicine:

## BLADDER TEA

4 tablespoons of dried nettle leaves
2 tablespoons of dried elderberries

2 tablespoons of dried primrose flowers

Mix everything well. Then take 2 teaspoons of the mixture and put them in a pot. Boil them for about 3 minutes with 2 cups of water. Then strain and drink sip by sip. You can also sweeten the tea with some honey.

Eating or drinking cranberries or cranberry juice also has a favorable effect.

A remedy that has been used in medicine since the 18th century is silver. It has been used in various forms as a remedy for epilepsy, inflammation, spasms, as well as diarrhea and stomach problems. Even today, it is beneficial for inflammation as colloidal silver in so-called silver water. One could also produce this oneself through electrolysis in water, but this is certainly not an old home remedy and is better left to professional hands.

## 27. BLADDER WEAKNESS, INCONTINENCE

Pumpkin is believed to help with bladder weakness in various forms. You can snack on pumpkin seeds, eat roasted pumpkin seeds, pumpkin vegetables, pumpkin compote, or pumpkin soup.

A good dose is 3 tablespoons of pumpkin seeds spread throughout the day.

Teas made from horsetail, goldenrod, nettles, cranberry leaves, and hops are also very helpful.

They are often used in combination. Herbal teas have been used as home remedies for bladder weakness. Here is an old recipe for a bladder weakness tea:

BLADDER WEAKNESS TEA 1

2 tablespoons of oak bark
2 tablespoons of knotweed herb
2 tablespoons of bearberry leaves
2 tablespoons of St. John's Wort

Mix everything well and pour 1 teaspoon of the mixture over 1 cup of boiling water, cover and let steep for 15 minutes, then strain. Drink up to 2 cups per day for up to 1 month.

All information and home remedies provided are for informational purposes only. They do not represent current scientific knowledge and are not intended for self-medication. Diagnosis and medication can only be carried out by a doctor or pharmacist.

Another tea for bladder weakness, which was consumed twice a day for up to 3 weeks:

## BLADDER WEAKNESS TEA 2

8 tablespoons of goldenrod
8 tablespoons of white dead-nettle
6 tablespoons of rose hips without seeds
4 tablespoons of horsetail
4 tablespoons of heather
2 tablespoons of marigold flowers
2 tablespoons of sage
2 tablespoons of rosemary

Use all dried herbs, mix well. Pour 1 teaspoon of the mixture over 1 cup of boiling water, cover and let steep for 10 minutes, then strain.

And another recipe for a tea that should be consumed 3 times a day for 1 month.

## BLADDER WEAKNESS TEA 3

10 tablespoons of lady's mantle herb
6 tablespoons of fennel seeds
6 tablespoons of willowherb herb

> Mix all dried herbs thoroughly. Brew 1 teaspoon of the herbal mixture with boiling water, cover and let steep for 10 minutes, then strain.

Especially for nocturnal bladder weakness, a tea made from dandelion roots, taken for one month, was recommended.

Other teas believed to have potential against bladder weakness include teas made from wormwood, nettle herb, yarrow, lemon balm, sage, and St. John's Wort.

Cranberry juice is also said to have a beneficial effect on bladder weakness.

## DANDELION ROOT TEA AGAINST BLADDER WEAKNESS

> In one liter of water, boil 2 tablespoons of dandelion root for 10 minutes, and drink one glass of it each morning.

## 28. ANEMIA

In spring, eating salad with dandelion, watercress, and lamb's lettuce is said to be a blood tonic.

Products made from animal offal help the blood because they contain iron.

Particularly, blood sausage is very rich in iron and was recommended for anemia.

A folk remedy was iron sugar, which was believed to help with anemia.

Beetroot and beetroot juice are good for the blood.

An old home remedy was also red wine with egg and honey.

## RED WINE WITH EGG AND HONEY

500 ml red wine

2 egg yolks

2 tablespoons honey

Mix everything well and heat slightly. It should be drunk daily before bedtime for a month.

## 29. HYPTERTENSION

Remedies for hypertension in the past included methods such as bloodletting, which was prescribed for various reasons, as well as the application of leeches and cupping therapy with cups.

It was known that exercise can help, especially when done in fresh air.

Garlic and onions have a positive effect on high blood pressure.

Some herbal tea blends were said to positively influence hypertension.

Particularly noteworthy are blends containing mistletoe and hawthorn, as well as arnica, hops, and valerian.

Onions, garlic, wild garlic, and horsetail can lower blood pressure.

Licorice raises blood pressure.

## 30. BLOOD PURIFICATION

Blood purification tincture should be consumed morning and evening, one cup each time.

## BLOOD PURIFICATION TINCTURE

500 g oat
100 g chicory root
6 g saltpeter
8 l water

Boil everything together and reduce to 4 liters. Then strain several times through a cloth for purification.

Drink 2 cups of blood purification tea per day.

## BLOOD PURIFICATION TEA

> 10 g heather
> 10 g parsley
> 10 g nettle root
> 10 g bloodroot with root
> 10 g dead-nettle with flower
> 10 g centaury with flower
> 3 g juniper
> 3 g buckthorn bark
> 1.5 g valerian
>
> Mix and pour 1 teaspoon of the mixture into a cup of boiling water. Drink 2 cups per day.
>
> You can also add strawberry leaves, raspberry leaves, blackberry leaves, wild pansy, blackthorn blossoms, and couchgrass roots.

Since the 17th century, it has been customary to eat water violet in salads for blood purification in the spring.

Consume dishes with lots of leek, onions, or garlic.

You can also eat garlic bread or onion bread.

Grate an apple, mix with raw egg, and consume once a week.

It is recommended to eat plenty of beetroot.

For centuries, it has been customary to undergo a birch sap cure at the beginning of spring or end of winter. Drink one cup of birch water in the morning and evening.

## 31. GANGRENE DISEASE

(formerly used unspecifically for bacterial or viral infections or infected hemorrhagic disorders resulting in tissue necrosis)

Apply compresses of bread and milk, cooked to a paste and wrapped in cloth, on the wound, and cover with a cloth spread with unsalted butter in case of suppuration.

Apply hot compresses with sliced and brewed carline thistle (Carlina vulgaris).

Apply compresses with cold water, towels wrapped in ice or snow.

## 32. NAUSEA

Ginger tea, chamomile tea, and peppermint tea are old home remedies for nausea.

If nausea occurs after breakfast, it is advisable to avoid acidic drinks such as apple juice, orange juice, etc., for breakfast.

## 33. BREAST SWELLING, BREAST TENSION

Feelings of tension in the breasts sometimes occur more frequently in women, especially before or during menopause.

Here, quark compresses or wraps, where quark is applied thickly on a cloth and placed around the breast, were popular.

Also, chaste tree seeds, which are now mostly known as monk's pepper, were popular and are still considered effective.

Consumption was done by chewing some seeds or as tea or tincture. Chaste tree was chewed by monks living in celibacy to suppress libido, hence the name.

## MONK'S PEPPER TEA

1 teaspoon of chaste tree seeds is poured over with a cup of boiling water and left covered for 10 minutes. Then strain. Drink up to 3 cups a day.

## MONK'S PEPPER TINCTURE

Pour 180 g of crushed chaste tree seeds into a glass with 1 liter of 40% alcohol spirits such as grain alcohol or vodka. Close the glass and let it sit warm for about a week, but not in the sun. Then strain and fill the tincture into dark bottles. A dose is about 20-30 drops of the tincture.

## 34. DECUBITUS, SEDES

Often change the lying position and wash with cold water.

Massage with oil, such as olive oil, calendula oil, or arnica oil.

## 35. CIRCULATION DISORDERS, COLD HANDS OR FEET

Tips here were to spend a lot of time outdoors, brush hands and feet with cold water, or take alternating baths.

Limbs should be massaged with pine oil.

## 36. DIARRHEA

Diarrhea due to fatty or excessive food intake can be combated by abstaining.

To support, only consume chicken broth and white bread and drink tea. A good red mulled wine with cinnamon and nutmeg can also help with diarrhea.

Others swear by a glass of Burgundy in the morning and evening.

Bananas, cocoa, and even bitter chocolate have constipating effects and could stop diarrhea.

Eating zwieback stops and halts diarrhea.

In France, barley decoction or almond milk was used against diarrhea. Almond milk was also the remedy of choice in southern Germany.

Even a cup of rye, roasted and ground, brewed like coffee, was a classic home remedy.

Even grated charcoal from softwoods or cork can stop diarrhea. Marshmallow root tea was a home remedy for diarrhea.

## MARSHMALLOW ROOT TEA

1 teaspoon marshmallow root with a cup of cold water and let it steep for 30 minutes.

Stir occasionally. Hot water destroys many active ingredients of the marshmallow root.

Chewing and eating dried blueberries or blackberries can help with diarrhea.

Also, psyllium husk is a home remedy, as well as tea from lady's mantle, willow leaves, or tormentil.

Drink tea made from blackberry leaves.

## BLACKBERRY LEAF TEA

2 teaspoons dried blackberry leaves infuse with 1 cup of boiling water, let it steep for 5 minutes, and strain.

Attached is a specific diarrhea tea.

## DIARRHEA TEA

> 1 tablespoon sage
> 1 tablespoon chamomile flowers
> 1 tablespoon oak bark
> 1 tablespoon gentian
>
> Mix everything well. Brew 1 teaspoon with a cup of boiling water, let it steep covered for 5 minutes, strain, and drink slowly.

Drink tea made from dried cherry stems. Stems from sour cherries should be particularly effective.

## TEA MADE FROM DRIED CHERRY STEMS

> 1 tablespoon dried cherry stems pour over with 1 cup of boiling water and let it steep covered for 15 minutes.

Drinking alant tea several times a day was helpful for diarrhea.

Drink rice water soup. This is an old French home remedy.

## RICE WATER SOUP

> 3 tablespoons rice cook in 500 ml of water until soft. The soup is not seasoned but eaten as it is.

Drink soup made from rye flour.

## RYE FLOUR SOUP

> 3 tablespoons rye flour boil in 500 ml of water for about 10 minutes. The soup is eaten unseasoned.

For diarrhea of any severity, oatmeal is recommended.

## OATMEAL

> 1 cup oatmeal soak in 1 liter of water for about 2 hours.
>
> Then cook for 1 hour. Half of this porridge is consumed in the morning for breakfast instead of coffee, after 2 hours the remainder is warmed up and drunk.

Also, the following diarrhea patch is said to help.

## DIARRHEA PATCH

> 3 tablespoons bread crust
> 2 tablespoons crushed juniper berries
> 1 tablespoon caraway seeds
> 1 tablespoon ginger
> 1 tablespoon cloves
> 1 tablespoon cinnamon
> 1 tablespoon nutmeg
> mix with warmed red wine or grain alcohol to form a paste. This is spread on leather and attached to the stomach or abdomen.

Boil some cinnamon in milk and drink.

Drink tea from the leaves or bark of the slippery elm.

### SLIPPERY ELM TEA

1 tablespoon slippery elm leaves, dried infuse with 1 cup of boiling water, let it steep covered for 5 minutes, and strain.

### ELM BARK TEA

1 teaspoon elm bark infuse with 1 cup of boiling water, let it steep covered for 5 minutes, and strain.

Also, teas made from cumin, fennel, anise, and chamomile may help to stop diarrhea.

Other remedies that work well against diarrhea are cooked carrots, bananas, grated apples, mashed potatoes, zwieback.

It was not until the early 20th century that carrot soup according to Moro became part of home remedies.

### MORO SOUP

500 g carrots
1 liter of water
3 g salt

> Peel the carrots, roughly chop them, and cook them in the water for at least one hour. Then strain or puree through a sieve.
> Now add 3 g of salt and fill up this carrot puree with boiled water again to 1 liter. The porridge should be administered in small portions. It is important for successful application that the carrots have been cooked for at least 1 hour!

## MORO SOUP, CHILD-FRIENDLY

> 500 g carrots
> 1 liter of water
> 1 splash of lemon
> 3 g salt
> 1 teaspoon butter
> 1 teaspoon sugar
>
> Peel the carrots, put everything in a pot, cook for about 1.5 hours, and process into a porridge.
> The splash of lemon ensures that the sugar contained in the carrots is better split. Butter and sugar improve the taste of the porridge slightly. This porridge should also be administered in small amounts.

Birch charcoal can also help against stomach cramps.

## BIRCH CHARCOAL

All information and home remedies provided are for informational purposes only. They do not represent current scientific knowledge and are not intended for self-medication. Diagnosis and medication can only be carried out by a doctor or pharmacist.

> 1/2 teaspoon powdered birch charcoal moisten with a little
> spirits or grain alcohol and take.

Cook the root of the mullein in red wine and drink the broth lukewarm.

## MULLEIN ROOT WINE

> 1 tablespoon mullein roots,
>
> crushed boil in 150 ml of red wine, let it cool, and drink lukewarm.

## 37. INFLAMMATION IN MOUTH AND THROAT

Gargling with chamomile tea was a proven home remedy.

## CHAMOMILE TEA

> Infuse 1-2 tablespoon of chamomile with boiling water and
> let it steep for 5 minutes. Gargling with herbal tea was also
> done several times a day.

Gargling with herbal tea was also done several times a day.

## HERBAL TEAFOR GARGLING

1 tablespoon peppermint leaves

1 tablespoon chamomile flowers

1 tablespoon rose petals

1 tablespoon sage

Infuse with a cup of boiling water, let it steep for 10 minutes, strain.

Sanicle tea, consumed or used for gargling, was a remedy for mouth inflammations.

## 38. INFLAMMATIONS

Chamomile has always been a popular home remedy for both internal and external inflammations. Chamomile tea was not only consumed but also used for gargling or bathing inflamed limbs, or making compresses or poultices for inflamed areas.

Marigold, mostly used as a salve, was applied to inflamed areas.

A simple remedy for mouth inflammations was also chewing a clove.

Inflamed joints were often wrapped in a poultice of oatmeal in milk. Nettles were also used for inflamed joints or muscles. Nettle tea and even eating nettles were believed to positively influence inflammations.

In case of finger inflammations, bathing in an oak bark decoction or oak bark tea was common.

Bathing in chamomile tea was also customary for inflammations.

Crushed larch needles were applied for inflammations to accelerate the healing process.

## 39. VOMITING

For vomiting, a compress with a cloth dipped in cold water around the neck and on the stomach, drinking cold water or strong coffee without milk, applying a mustard plaster on the stomach, or taking a warm foot bath were recommended.

Drinking saltwater, adding 1 tsp of salt to 1 glass of water, is also advisable.

Drinking warm water with butter or olive oil should also help.

A remedy for vomiting, occurring after meals, is an anti-emetic powder.

ANTI-EMETIC POWDER

2 tbsp ground ginger
2 tbsp ground cumin
2 tbsp salt

Mix everything well. Take 1 tsp of this powder after meals for about 1 week.

Taking licorice charcoal should also help.

As early as the 18th century, vanilla ice cream was recommended for pregnant women suffering from vomiting.

Other folk remedies to stop vomiting included fresh milk, fresh oysters, and raw egg yolk.

## 40. FROSTBITE

For frostbite, compresses made from grated turnips or ice-cold sauerkraut can alleviate discomfort.

Frozen areas can be washed with warm brandy.

Rubbing with camphor spirit should also help.

In England, it was common to make compresses with cloths dipped in warm vinegar for frostbites and chilblains.

Compresses with warm oak leaf decoction were also common.

## 41. PREVENT FROSTBITE

To prevent frostbite, thickly apply fat, cream, or ointment to vulnerable limbs and skin areas.

If the limbs become very cold and frostbite is imminent, rub them with snow or ice-cold water until blood circulation returns.

Avoid drinking alcoholic beverages in the cold. Hot drinks can be very helpful.

When it's very cold, keep moving to prevent frostbite, don't stand still, don't sit and rest, as you might be overcome by sleep, followed by death.

In case of frostbite, apply lentil ointment to the affected areas overnight. Rinse the areas well in the morning.

## LENTILOINTMENT

Dry and crush brown lentils. Mix the lentil flour with lard.

Compresses made from grated horseradish and hot water were another home remedy.

## 42. COLD WITH FLU-LIKE INFECTION

Colds come with various symptoms such as cough, runny nose, sore throat, etc. You can find additional home remedies for these symptoms under the respective headings.

Resting in bed with a sweat treatment, preferably with a scarf around the neck, could shorten the duration of the cold.

A commonly used home remedy, especially among male rural populations in the south, was to heat up a double shot of fruit brandy with a pinch of pepper and drink it hot.

Drinking hot lemon water is also helpful as a preventive measure.

Eucalyptus oil was inhaled in hot water.

A mixture of eucalyptus oil and other ingredients was rubbed on the chest and back.

## EUCALYPTU-LAVENDER CHEST BALM

- 100 ml almond oil
- 15 drops eucalyptus oil
- 15 drops lavender oil

Mix everything well and rub it on the chest and back, then wrap with a cloth.

## HOT LEMON

Squeeze the juice of a lemon into water heated to about 60°C, and drink with or without sugar or honey.

inden flower tea with some honey is an old home remedy for colds.

## LINDEN FLOWER TEA

1-2 teaspoons dried linden flowers
Pour one cup boiling water over the dried linden flowers and let steep for 5-10 minutes, then strain. The tea can also be sweetened with 1 tablespoon of honey.

Another home remedy is hot elderberry juice with some honey.

ELDERBERRY JUICE

1 kg ripe elderberries
1 liter water

Put the water and elderberries in a pot, bring to a boil, and simmer until the berries are soft. Strain through a sieve or cloth, pressing the berries well. Consume as much as possible throughout the day.

To preserve the juice, you can can it in bottles or jars.

You can also add the juice of 1/2 lemon per liter of juice and mix it with 200 g of sugar. Then, bring it to a boil again and fill it hot into bottles or jars, seal them, and store them in a dark place.

In spring, tea made from spruce shoots is highly recommended.

SPRUCE TEA

- A handful of fresh spruce shoots

> - 500 ml water
>   Pour boiling water over the spruce shoots and let steep covered for 20 minutes, then drink as hot as possible.

You can also use hot tea made from spruce tip syrup or pine tip syrup.

## SPRUCE SYRUP OR PINE SYRUP

> - Spruce tips or pine tips, freshly picked in spring
> - water
>
> Wash the tips well with water to remove dirt and pollen. Cover generously with water, add a sliced lemon, and weigh down with a plate to ensure all tips are well covered with liquid. Let it sit overnight. Then slowly simmer until the tips lose their color. Let it steep for at least another 10 hours. Strain the liquid through a sieve or cloth and squeeze the tips well. Weigh the liquid and mix it with an equal amount of sugar, then simmer for another 5 minutes. Fill the syrup into prepared jars or bottles and seal tightly
> The syrup is very concentrated and can be diluted up to 1:10.

Sage tea is a home remedy for colds.

## SAGE TEA

> - 2 teaspoons dried sage leaves
>
>   Pour boiling water over the leaves, let steep covered for 10 minutes, then strain. Sage tea can be consumed hot or cold.

Elderflower tea has been used for centuries as a remedy for colds and runny noses. You can also inhale the steam.

## ELDERFLOWER TEA

> - 2 teaspoons dried or fresh elderflowers
>
>   Pour one cup boiling water over the dried elderflowers and let steep for 5 minutes.

Drinking a sweat-inducing tea and sweating in bed is an old home remedy.

## SWEATING TEA

> - 10 g linden flowers
> - 10 g elder flowers
> - 10 g yarrow
> - 10 g nettles
> - 5 g sage
> - 5 g wormwood

> Mix all dried herbs well. Brew 1 tablespoon of this mixture with 250 ml boiling water, cover and let steep for 10 minutes.

Below is an old recipe for a fever tea:

## FEVERTEA FOR COLD

- 10 g centaury
- 10 g yarrow
- 10 g columbine
- 10 g shepherd's purse
- 5 g marigold
- 5 g poplar leaves

Mix all herbs well and brew 1 tablespoon with 250 ml boiling water, cover and let steep for 10 minutes. Use twice a day.

Another very old home remedy for fever and colds is raisin tea.

## RAISIN TEA

- 1 cupof raisins
- 2 liters of water

Put the raisins and water in a pot, bring to a boil, and simmer until the raisins are soft. Strain through a sieve

and press the raisins well. Drink as much as possible
throughout the day.

Warming calf compresses with linen towels dipped in warm water can alleviate discomfort.

Also, for centuries, people have used onion socks:

## ONION SOCK

Peel and finely slice 2 onions, sauté them in butter, place them on two cloths, and bind these as hot as possible to the soles of the feet.

Another remedy involving onions was to place a sliced onion next to the bed, near the head. The onion vapors were believed to help reduce swollen nasal passages.

Oatmeal gruel was also given as a light diet supplement.

## OATMEAL GRUEL

- 100 g oat flakes
- 500 ml water

Boil the oat flakes in water and simmer for several minutes. Then add a pinch of salt.

## 43. FEVER

Restricting physical activities and, if possible, bed rest are the best home remedies for fever. One of the oldest remedies for fever and inflammation was barley gruel, which was already known by Hippocrates. Today, it would be seen as a therapeutic diet. As a German version of the tisane, barley porridge could be considered.

### BARLEY PORRIDGE

100 ml crushed barley is boiled with 1 liter of water until the barley is fully swollen and the grains burst. Then, some vinegar or sour honey (oxymel) was added. Either the water was strained, squeezed, and drunk cold, or the barley was eaten.

Sour honey was a remedy of ancient Romans. The name oxymel for sour honey derives from the Latin 'oxymeli' (sour and honey). Sour honey was not only a remedy for fever but also for many other illnesses, depending on the herbs used.

### SOUR HONEY

> Mix 4 tbsp forest honey with 1 tbsp wine vinegar, pour
> into a bottle, remove all air bubbles, and seal.
> Depending on the diseases to be treated, herbs, roots,
> or flowers were added.

A particularly common home remedy for fever in southern Germany and Austria was salep. Salep itself has been used since ancient times and entered Germany in the 15th century. Salep consists of the dried tubers of orchids (various species of orchids such as Common Spotted Orchid, Greater Butterfly Orchid, Leopard Marsh Orchid, and Pyramidal Orchid

## SALEP DRINK

> 3 g salep is boiled in 1 liter of water for 15 minutes and
> then given as a drink.

During fever, strict bed rest was usually observed.

It was always important to reduce high fever to spare the circulation and body. The simplest means to do this were calf compresses. These were often made with cold water alone, but also with a water-vinegar solution consisting of 500 ml water and 100 ml wine vinegar.

Common teas included lime blossom tea, chamomile tea, thyme tea, elderflower tea, peppermint tea.

## FIVER TEA 1

- 20 g chopped ginger
- 10 g ried elderflower
- 10 g dried peppermint

Pour over with 2 cups of boiling water, let steep covered for 10 minutes, strain. Drink a maximum of 5 cups per day.

## FIVER TEA 2

- 2 tbsp dried rose hips, seedless
- 3 tbsp elderflowers
- 2 tbsp dried elderberries
- 3 tbsp lime blossoms
- 2 tbsp yarrow

Pour 1 tbsp of the mixture over 1 cup of boiling water, let steep for 10 minutes, strain, and drink slowly while hot.

If those with fever were plagued by intense thirst, they were often given hawthorn juice or barberry juice.

## 44. PSORIASIS

One home remedy was to apply egg white to the psoriasis patches in the morning for 30 minutes and then wash it off.

Sulfur baths for the affected areas were also recommended.

To support healing, sarsaparilla root tea should be consumed.

### SARSAPARILLA ROOT TEA

1 teaspoon of sarsaparilla root infused in one cup of boiling water for 10 minutes, then strained.

## 45. SKIN LICHEN

For lichens, our ancestors often recommended frequent washings with soap water or salt water.

Another home remedy is to moisten the lichen often with sulfur water.

Washings with a decoction of horseradish leaves, bran, onions, or garlic were also used.

Roots of common sorrel were grated and mixed with butter or lard. In the morning and evening, the lichens were coated with this mixture.

Maintaining a diet consisting mainly of plant-based foods, avoiding smoked or heavily salted foods, as well as pork, brandy, or beer is recommended.

Lichens often have their origin in a weakened body, so strengthening the body's defenses is important.

The outermost skin of dandelion leaves was removed and placed on the lichen.

For beard lichen, a decoction of horsetail is said to have been effective. This can be used as a compress or the area can be bathed or dabbed with it.

Compresses with fresh or steeped comfrey leaves as well as washings with a decoction of boiled comfrey leaves were believed to make lichens disappear.

## 46. SPOTS, BRUISES, HEMATOMAS

Immediately after the blow or injury, bandages should prevent the appearance of bruises.

Cooling and cold compresses were also preferred methods.

Arnica, as a tea, ointment, or compress, was a remedy for bruises.

## ARNICA COMPRESS

Infuse 2 teaspoons of arnica in 1 cup of hot water, let it steep for 5 minutes, then strain. Moisten a linen cloth with it and apply it to the affected area. Change it frequently.

Placing a linen cloth soaked in brandy should dispel the bruise. A cloth soaked in vinegar should also help. It was also recommended to place a halved onion with the cut side on the skin.

Massaging with St. John's Wort oil can disperse the spots.

## 47. BOILS, CARBUNCLES

An old remedy is to drink nettle tea.

## NETTLE TEA

- 1-2 teaspoons of nettle herb, finely cut
  Infuse with one cup of boiling water and let it steep for about 4 minutes.

Avoid drinking alcohol, refrain from pork and pork offal.

Avoid heavily spiced dishes.

Apply cabbage leaf compresses to the affected areas, removing the ribs from the cabbage leaves, then roll them soft with a rolling pin, apply them to the affected area, and tie them with a bandage.

Bathe the affected areas with chamomile tea.

Daisy compresses were also an old home remedy.

## DAISY COMPRESS

Boil 100 g of daisy flowers in 500 ml of water for a few minutes. Then soak a linen cloth with the decoction and apply it to the affected area. Repeat this several times.

A comfrey compress should also help.

## COMFREY COMPRESS

Cook some crushed leaves of the comfrey plant in a little water or milk. Place the leaves still warm directly on the affected area. Repeat several times.

Mix cereal porridge with chamomile and apply it as a compress or plaster.

To relieve pain, administer warm and cold vinegar compresses.

## 48. ATHLET'S FOOT

An old home remedy is to crush garlic and apply the garlic paste several times a day.

Applying the affected areas with St. John's Wort oil or lavender oil should help against athlete's foot.

Peppermint, tea tree oil, and myrrh were also remedies used against athlete's foot. The concentrated essential oils were usually applied diluted with olive oil. You can spread it on your feet or use it in foot baths.

## 49. FOOT SWEAT

You should take cold foot baths more often. Also, alternating baths, with the first and last being cold, could be helpful.

Foot baths with mustard flour or even with caraway were also recommended.

## 50. GALLSTONES

Eat lots of vegetables cooked in meat broth, chicory, endive, parsley, red cabbage, chervil, etc., then juicy fruits: cherries, strawberries, mulberries, gooseberries, raspberries in large quantities, also drink whey sweetened with honey in spring, eat 3-4 egg yolks daily to expel the stones.

For gallstone colic, the intake of 1 tablespoon of lemon juice in chamomile tea or almond oil was recommended. After that, a glass of whey or water should be drunk.

## 51. MEMORY ENHANCEMENT

Practice makes perfect! Engaging activities that challenge the brain prevent deterioration. Games, puzzles, and memory exercises are preventive.

Some also rely on herbal remedies - especially ginkgo and ginseng are central to the effort.

Some foods are also believed to enhance brain and memory performance. Notably, walnuts, carrots, flaxseed oil, and cabbage are mentioned. Woodruff tea can enhance concentration.

WOODRUFF TEA

---

> Infuse 1 teaspoon of woodruff with one cup of boiling water. Let it steep for 15 minutes covered, strain, and drink.

## 52. JOINT PAIN

One should avoid overloading the joints with joint pain.

In the past, bloodletting and treatment with leeches were home remedies.

Elevating the affected joint provides relief.

Fruits and vegetables, fish, nuts, and grain products are considered positively influential, whereas pork is considered negative.

Warm and cold mud baths are helpful and have been documented since Roman times.

Baths with the addition of sulfur-containing preparations or ointments with sulfur are helpful home remedies.

A widely used home remedy in earlier days was camphor. Painful joints were rubbed with camphor tincture or ointment.

Cabbage wraps were common.

Tinctures and ointments made from devil's claw have been used for a long time.

Salve made from arnica or marigold was also a common home remedy for painful joints.

Massaging with caraway oil was common for joint pain.

Rubbing with rosemary tincture should help with joint pain.

## ROSEMARY TINCTURE

Fill rosemary into a sealable glass and press it down so that the glass is half full. Then fill it up with high-proof (>=40%) alcohol, close it, and let it stand in a warm place for 3 weeks, shaking it daily. Then strain, squeeze out the herb, fill the liquid into dark bottles, and seal them well.

Applying willow bark extract should also help. This should also be very helpful for arthritis and inflammatory joint problems. You can also apply willow bark compresses. These should be particularly helpful for joint pain.

## WILLOW BARK EXTRACT

Fill crushed willow bark into a sealable glass and press it down so that the glass is half full. Then fill it up with high-proof alcohol (preferably >=50%), close it, and let it stand in a warm place for 3 weeks, shaking it daily. Then strain, squeeze out the herb, fill the liquid into dark bottles, and seal them well.

Quark compresses were, like mustard compresses for joint pain, a preferred home remedy..

## MUSTARD COMPRESS

4-5 tablespoons of crushed mustard seeds are mixed with some water to form a paste, which is then applied to a clean linen cloth. This cloth is placed on the affected area. A mustard poultice should only be left on for a few minutes (2-5 minutes), and after getting used to it, the time can be extended slightly. It should also be applied for a maximum of 5 days.

Comfrey was also a preferred remedy. Ointments or tinctures were made from comfrey. But compresses with comfrey were also common.

## COMFREY POULTICE

Grind about 3 tablespoons of comfrey root and mix it with some hot water to form a paste. Apply this warm paste onto a cloth and wrap it around the joint. This compress can be renewed every 3 hours.

## 53. IRRITABILITY

To combat irritability, one can drink valerian tea, hops tea, or peppermint tea. Valerian tea should be consumed in a maximum of 2 cups per day.

## CALERIAN TEA

2 teaspoons of valerian root in 250 ml of cold water and let it steep for 12 hours. Stir occasionally.

## VALERIANTEA ASAHOT INFUSION

1 teaspoon of valerian root pour over 500 ml of boiling water, cover, and let steep for 15 minutes, then strain.

## HOPS TEA

1 teaspoon of hops flowers or cones, dried pour over 250 ml of boiling water and let it steep for 10 minutes, then strain. Drink in small sips.

## PEPPERMINT TEA

> 1-2 teaspoons of dried peppermint leaves pour over
> 250 ml of boiling water and let it steep for 5-10
> minutes, then strain.

You can also drink a mixture of valerian root and lemon balm leaves.

## VALERIAN-LEMON BALM TEA

> 1 teaspoon of valerian root
> 1 teaspoon of lemon balm leaves
> brew with 250 ml of boiling water and let steep
> covered for 15 minutes. Then strain.

## 54. BARLEYCORN

You can rinse the eye with eyebright tea with a little salt.

Apply chamomile tea compresses filtered multiple times through a cloth to the barleycorn.

Long ago, warm poultices made from bread, milk, and saffron were common.

Apply a piece of raw onion or honey cake dough with onions.

In the morning, dab the barleycorn before eating with saliva or urine.

Another home remedy is to soak a bun in hot milk, wrap it in a cloth, and then place it on the closed eye.

## 55. GOUT

For gout, a simple diet was followed, avoiding hot beverages and heavily spiced foods.

Consuming plenty of strawberries is said to help during acute attacks.

A mixed tea of green and black tea, sweetened with honey, is believed to alleviate gout.

Drinking ginger with milk daily is thought to reduce symptoms.

Good King Henry (chenopodium bonus-henricus) was applied to the gouty areas of the feet and secured with a bandage.

Rubbing with comfrey oil or angelica root oil was believed to provide relief to those suffering from gout.

A mixture of chamomile oil with a little brandy for rubbing is also recommended. Afterwards, the affected limbs were wrapped in hot towels.

For foot gout (podagra), the following remedy, applied every 12 hours, is said to be helpful:

## RICE-YEAST COMPRESS

- • 500 g rice flour
- • 50 g brewer's yeast
- • 30 g salt

All ingredients are mixed to form a thick dough. This is applied to the soles of the feet and wrapped with flannel or linen. Wash off with bran and brandy in warm soapy water.

Another recommended compress was a paste made from mashed beech ash, mashed birch leaves, coltsfoot leaves, and castor leaves, wrapped in a cloth and tied to the gouty limb.

A folk remedy for gout was also a drink made from mustard and wine, of which a glass was consumed early in the morning, followed by spending a few hours in bed sweating.

## MUSTARD-WINE

50 g ground black mustard mixed with 1 liter of white wine in a bottle, sealed, and left to stand in a warm place for 4 days. Then strain and store in a dark bottle in a cool place.

## GINGER MILK

Add 1 teaspoon of powdered ginger to a glass of hot milk. The milk can also be sweetened with a little honey or sugar.

To minimize the pain of a gout attack, the area should be rubbed with bacon.

After a gout attack, a mustard seed paste was applied to the gouty limb or bags of warmed bean flour were applied.

Taking cod liver oil from fish is believed to help alleviate gout symptoms.

Stockings made of dog hair were believed to help with gout.

## GOUT AND RHEUMATISM TEA

3 tablespoons of birch leaves
3 tablespoons of nettle leaves
3 tablespoons of buckthorn bark

Pour 1 teaspoon each with boiling water, let it steep for 10 minutes, and strain. The tea can be sweetened with a little honey. Drink one cup twice daily.

## 56. INFLUENZA

For influenza, strict bed rest with sweating and plenty of sleep was the first choice home remedy.

To induce sweating, warm or hot beer was consumed, with or without honey.

To further support sweating, a hot stone or hot water bottle was placed in bed.

Inhalation with essential oils such as peppermint oil, eucalyptus oil, or chamomile tea was common.

Cold compresses on the calves were used for fever.

One of the most effective remedies was considered to be hot peppermint tea, especially when consumed in the evening.

## 57. HAIR LOSS, HAIR GROWTH PROMOTION

Birch water has long been believed to have a positive effect on hair loss. Simply massage birch water into the scalp after washing the hair and do not rinse it out. But even without birch water, scalp massage is a good way to address hair loss and promote circulation.

Walnuts are also believed to be good for hair loss. You can eat walnuts, but you can also wash your hair with a walnut leaf decoction. To do this, add about 5 leaves to a liter of water and simmer for 5 minutes. Then wash the hair with it after shampooing and rinsing, and massage it into the scalp. This decoction may also darken the hair - caution is advised with light-colored hair.

Washing with herbal decoctions can also be helpful. Suitable herbs include parsley, watercress, nasturtium, and thyme. Either infuse the herbs with boiling water and massage the liquid into the hair or scalp after washing, or prepare a tincture to massage into the scalp. If using infused herbs, you can also add a splash of vinegar.

The leaves of birch and boxwood, boiled in water for several minutes, can also be used for hair washing or as a hair tonic for subsequent massage.

An old home remedy for hair growth is to use a nettle hair treatment.

## NETTLE HAIR TREATMENT

- 500 g nettle leaves
- 1 liter water
- 1 liter white winegar

Boil all the ingredients in a pot and simmer for 30 minutes. Let it cool and use it for hair washing. Then

wrap the damp head with a towel and let it work
overnight.

As a hair tonic, rubbing alcohol with onions was also used. This
was massaged into the scalp daily.

## RUBBING ALCOHOL HAIR TINCTURE

Dice or chop 1 onion and place it in a glass with 100
ml of rubbing alcohol. Seal the glass and keep it warm
for 14 days. Shake it every day. Then strain it. The
tincture is then diluted with 300 ml of water, poured
into dark bottles, and sealed.

To strengthen hair growth, the head was also washed with oak
bark decoction. Caution: This decoction darkens the hair! It
was also a dye for gray dark hair.

Cardamom was considered a remedy for hair loss by the
Romans.

The head was washed with a cardamom decoction made from
seeds or the herb.

Castor oil, massaged into the scalp, was also considered a
remedy for hair loss.

## 58. HAIR PROBLEMS

If the hair no longer shines as it should, it was treated with lime blossom tea for some time. This was massaged into the hair after washing and not rinsed out.

Massaging the scalp with a concentrated nettle decoction was also believed to ensure strong and beautiful hair. This decoction was massaged into the hair after washing and not rinsed out.

## NETTLE DECOCTION

Boil 500 g nettle herb in 500 ml water briefly and let it cool. Then strain it.

For oily hair, washing with horsetail tea was believed to help.

Very thin hair was supposed to be helped by an egg-olive oil treatment. For this, olive oil was mixed with an egg yolk (this makes mayonnaise!) and massaged into the hair about 1 hour before washing. This mayonnaise treatment was supposed to give shine and promote thicker hair growth.

In times when hair was not washed too often and unpleasant odors were covered with fragrant perfume, oily hair was powdered. Normal powders were used for this, but also simple flour. Delicious, surely not.

A beer rinse after washing the hair is believed to strengthen the hair and give it a beautiful shine. The beer should be left on for about 10 minutes and then rinsed out.

## 59. SORE THROAT, PHARYNGITIS

A simple remedy is gargling with salt water. To do this, add 1 tbsp of salt to a glass of warm water and gargle with it. Repeat gargling as needed.

During the waning moon, it is recommended to gargle with linden flower tea, while during the waxing moon, gargling with warm beer is advised.

Another home remedy was to bind a previously worn sock around the neck overnight for sore throats and swollen tonsils, and gargle with sage tea with honey.

In the evening, it is recommended to hold a cup of chamomile tea in the mouth in small sips before swallowing.

For pharyngitis, Sanicle tea was drunk or used for gargling. Also, elderflower tea, sage tea, marshmallow root tea, yarrow tea, thyme tea, mallow tea, and plantain tea are said to be helpful.

### MARSHMALLOW ROOT TEA

1 tsp marshmallow root is boiled in a large cup of water for 3 minutes. Then strain and drink hot.

### HOARSENESS TEA

1 tsp marshmallow root is boiled with 1 tsp grated or sliced ginger in a large cup of water for 3 minutes. Then, add 1 tsp peppermint leaves to a cup and pour

the hot infusion over it. Let it steep covered for another 5 minutes, then strain.

Daily intake of 2 tbsp of onion juice is considered an old home remedy for sore throats.

## ONION JUICE

Peel and chop 1 onion, sprinkle with honey or sugar, and let it sit for several hours. Take the juice tablespoon by tablespoon. The glass can be left, and more juice will form over time.

Another application for sore throats is onion milk.

## ONION MILK

Dice 2 onions and boil them with two cups of water. Let the infusion cool slightly until drinkable, then stir in 1 tbsp of honey and drink.

As a home remedy, honey and rock candy were dissolved in hot water and consumed in small sips.

Also, hot elderberry juice, hot linden flower tea, and steam baths with chamomile are old home remedies.

## CHAMOMILE STEAM BATH

> Infuse 3 tsp of chamomile in a pot with 500 ml of
> boiling water. Lean over the pot as hot as possible,
> covering your head and the pot with a cloth.

Wraps with hayflowers around the neck were often applied, especially in rural areas in the south.

## HAYFLOWER WRAP

> Hayflowers are the dried plants growing on a flowering meadow.
>
> For a wrap, wrap the meadow hay in a cloth and steam it in water vapor in a pot for about 20 minutes, then wrap it around the affected body part.

Chewing a clove is said to help with throat inflammation.

An overnight wrap with warm quark, covered with a cloth, should alleviate sore throat.

## 60. HEMORRHOIDS

An old remedy to soothe hemorrhoids was steam baths. Boiling water was poured into a chamber pot, and one would sit on it. Sometimes wheat bran or cabbage leaves were added to the water.

In the 18th century, a salve made from Great Snapdragon (Antirrhinum majus) was used, where the whole herb was cooked in lard.

A decoction of oak bark, applied as a compress or poultice, was also said to help.

Flea Knotweed (Persicaria maculosa), formerly known as hemorrhoid herb in many regions, was drunk as a tea for hemorrhoids.

Tea made from Speedwell, Goldenrod, Ground Ivy, and Rose petals was also believed to be helpful.

Painful hemorrhoids were soothed with compresses made from teas of Yarrow, Red Clover, or Chamomile flowers.

For nodules, warm abdominal wraps were made, and Chamomile tea was consumed.

For sensitive or itchy nodules, almond oil was applied.

For painful nodules, leeches could be applied, followed by grated carrots.

## ANT STEAM BATH

he following old home remedy is likely to strongly conflict with conservation principles, as ants are protected. One would collect an anthill from the forest, including ants, eggs, etc., place it in a bucket at home,

and pour boiling water over it. Then, one would place
a board over the bucket, undress, and sit with the
naked buttocks on the board. The lower body and the
bucket would be covered with a dense cloth. After a
short time, the pain would improve.

For bleeding and discharges caused by hemorrhoids, one would drink Bittercress or Feverfew tea. Sharp foods and drinks as well as physical exertion should be avoided.

## BITTERCRESS TEA

1 tsp Bittercress
pour 1 cup of boiling water over it and let it steep
covered for 5-10 minutes. Then strain.

## 61. HAND CARE

There have always been many tips and tricks in the realm of home remedies for hand care. Especially during heavy work, hand care is important because who wants hands worn out and calloused, even though they attest to honest work and effort?

After cleaning and heavy work, hands were often moisturized with udder cream.

Also, soaking the hands in a mixture of a few drops of olive oil and warm milk made them attractive and soft again.

Another home remedy was soaking the hands in a mixture of olive oil and lemon juice, sometimes with a little honey added.

Cracked or chapped hands were also simply moisturized with butter.

## 62. URINARY BURNING

A diet with strong green or black tea diluted with cold water and sugar was a home remedy for urinary burning in Bavaria.

Drinking plenty of green tea was also the preferred method.

Drinking flaxseed tea was also common. In France, a shot of almond syrup was added to it.

FLAXSEED TEA

- 1-2 tsp whole flaxseeds

To prepare flaxseed tea, use cold water. Pour the seeds into a cup of cold water, let them steep for at least 20 minutes, stirring occasionally. Strain and drink the tea slightly warmed.

Local milk baths on the genitals were also used as a home remedy.

Marshmallow tea was also believed to be effective.

## 63. SKIN, WRINKLES

Skin wrinkles, especially those on the face, have bothered women for centuries.

There are many old home remedies used to reduce wrinkles. Birch leaf tea and garlic milk were believed to positively influence skin wrinkles.

Salves such as horse chestnut salve were also thought to be beneficial and minimize wrinkles.

A mask made from crushed strawberries and egg whites applied to the affected areas and left on for 10 minutes was particularly used for facial wrinkles.

A mask made from cottage cheese and honey was also believed to be helpful.

Various masks were also used, such as an apple-honey mask.

APPLE-HONEY MASK

> Grate an apple and mix it with 1 tbsp honey. Apply this mixture to your face for 10 minutes, then wash it off.

As a simpler alternative, you can also place apple slices or cucumber slices on specific areas of your face, such as the eyes, for 10-15 minutes.

## BARLEY HONEY MASK

> - 3 egg white
> - 1 tablespoon honey
> - 40 g barley flour
>
> Whisk the egg whites into stiff peaks and mix well with the honey and flour. Apply a thick layer of this mixture as a mask on the face and leave it on for 30 minutes. Then rinse off thoroughly with warm water.

Steam baths with chamomile tea or lime blossom tea were also used.

## 64. IMPURE SKIN

A steam bath with elderflower tea, chamomile tea, or even with hot water is helpful for acne-prone skin.

Among the Romans, mustard powder mixed with water was used as a skin cleanser for acne-prone skin.

## 65. SKIN INFLAMMATION

Applying calendula ointment to affected areas remains a preferred remedy to this day, just like using aloe vera ointment.

## 66. SKIN MARKS

Skin spots and age spots can be rubbed with lemon juice; they are said to become lighter as a result. You can also halve a lemon and dab the spots with the cut surface three times a day.

They can also be rubbed with a halved garlic clove.

A compress of freshly grated horseradish, applied for up to 30 minutes, is also said to help with spots.

The same effect is also attributed to cucumber juice. Grate and squeeze a cucumber. Soak a linen cloth in it and leave it on the spots for at least 20 minutes.

A traditional recipe from the south is also the spot paste; apply it to the spots and leave it on for 30 minutes.

SPOT PASTE

- 80 g cleavers
- 10 g dried and ground ginger

> - 10 g rose petals
>
> Mix everything together well and stir into a paste with
> 1 tbsp hot water.

A spot paste made from egg, curd, and magnesium sulfate is said to lighten or make age spots disappear. Cover the spots with the paste and leave it on for at least 10 minutes. Then rinse off with warm water.

## STAIN PASTE

> Mix 2 eggs with 100 g curd, 1 tbsp cream, and 1 tsp
> magnesium sulfate and beat until foamy.

Parsley juice, squeezed from fresh parsley, is said to lighten the spots when dabbed onto them.

## 67. SKINITCH

Baths with a mixture of milk and water followed by rubbing with olive oil have been a traditional home remedy in folk medicine since ancient times.

Salt baths can be helpful. Dissolve 50 g of salt per 10 liters of warm water and bathe in it for about 20 minutes. You can bathe only the affected body parts as needed or take a full bath with this saltwater. Afterwards, apply oil generously to the areas. Olive oil can be used, or herbal oils such as St. John's Wort oil.

Washing with a vinegar-water mixture is also recommended to provide relief.

A strict diet, avoiding meat, especially pork, was also advised.

A compress with horsetail was said to be helpful.

## HORSETAIL COMPRESS

You put 2 handfuls of horsetail into a liter of water and let it boil for 10 minutes. Then strain it, let it cool slightly, soak a cloth in it, and apply it to the affected areas.

Not too old of a home remedy: When the skin itches, apply crushed banana to it - this has proven particularly effective for dry skin.

Also, compresses with quark, applied directly to the skin and covered with a cloth, can be helpful.

Compresses with green or black tea were also practiced. Neurodermatitis and eczema were treated in this way as well.

## TEA ENVELOPE

For each cup of boiling water, use 2 heaping teaspoons of tea. Pour the boiling water over the tea and let it steep covered for 5 minutes. Then strain it, dip a cloth into it, and apply it to the affected areas. Let the tea work for about 10 minutes.

Wraps with wine vinegar, apple vinegar, or lemon, diluted with water, were common.

Essential oils such as tea tree oil, juniper berry oil, or rosemary oil could help. Wraps or baths can be used for this purpose.

## 68. HOARSENESS

Consuming a fresh egg yolk mixed with sugar on an empty stomach in the morning was widespread in many households.

Also, a mixture of garlic-honey taken in the morning and evening, 1 teaspoon to 1 tablespoon each, was considered to alleviate hoarseness.

### GARLIC HONEY

Crush the garlic, squeeze out the juice, and mix it with honey.

Also, warm radish or beetroot juice with sugar or honey, taken teaspoon by teaspoon throughout the day, was considered a good remedy for hoarseness.

### RADISH JUICE

> Grate or cut the radish into small pieces. Mix with sugar or honey and let it juice. Squeeze out the juice after a few hours.
>
> Beet juice can be prepared in the same way.

Linseed tea is a traditional remedy for hoarseness.

Other herbal teas have proven effective for hoarseness, such as teas made from mallow leaves, marshmallow root, coltsfoot, thyme, sage, or marshmallow root.

## COLTSFOOT TEA

> 2 teaspoons of coltsfoot leaves are poured over with a cup of boiling water and allowed to steep covered for 10 minutes. Then strain. You can drink up to 3 cups of it per day.

## 69. HERPES, COLD SORES

 key home remedy: Avoid disgust! Herpes is colloquially known as "disgust blisters," as intense disgust could trigger a herpes outbreak.

Avoiding stress also helps prevent a herpes outbreak.

Dab the cold sores with lemon balm tea or a piece of freshly cut ginger.

A remedy from not too distant times is to cover the area with toothpaste at the onset of the tingling sensation associated with herpes.

## 70. HEART AND CIRCULATION

Garlic, onion, and especially wild garlic when eaten raw, strengthen the circulation and heart. In the past, in some regions, "onion bread" or "garlic bread" was eaten. A slice of bread was spread with butter and topped with chopped or grated garlic or onions. The garlic or onions were also sautéed in a pan with a little oil.

An old home remedy is to drink milk with honey in the evening.

For many, a daily glass of red wine was also considered a heart-strengthening remedy.

Mistletoe tea was also used to strengthen the circulation and heart. This was prepared as a cold infusion with water.

Hawthorn as a tea or tincture is also an old remedy to strengthen the heart and circulation.

In some regions, clay compresses were made by spreading cold clay about 1 cm thick on the chest and covering it with a clean cloth; after about 20 minutes, the clay was washed off.

Plenty of exercise in the fresh air and also Russian steam baths in the Banja/Sauna strengthen the circulation and heart.

There are also various teas and herbal blends such as hawthorn tea, which were traditionally used to strengthen the heart and for heart complaints.

## HEART TEA 1

- 50 g savory
- 50 g lemon balm
- 50 g lime blossom
- 20 g hyssop
- 10 g anise

Mix everything well. Pour 1 teaspoon of the tea mixture with a cup of boiling water, let it steep for 10 minutes, strain. It can be consumed as is, or sweetened with some honey. This tea was consumed over 2-3 weeks, three times a day.

## HEART TINCTURE

- 20 g valerian root
- 15 g St. John's wort
- 15 g lemon balm
- 30 g passionflower herb
- 25 g ops cones

> Place everything in a glass and pour 700ml of spirits
> with at least 40% alcohol content (vodka, fruit brandy,
> grain spirits) over it, seal the glass, and let it stand in a
> warm place for 14 days. Then strain and fill into a
> brown bottle. Drink 1 tablespoon or take it in water.

## 71. HEART PALPITATIONS

Crushed lemon balm leaves were placed on the chest to alleviate heart palpitations.

Drinking apple juice in small sips throughout the day is said to calm heart palpitations.

Pouring lavender flowers with sugar water and taking it spoon by spoon was also an old folk medicine remedy.

## 72. LUMBAGO

The affected areas were rubbed with marigold ointment or arnica oil.

For lumbago, or when experiencing "lower back pain," many people often rubbed with rubbing alcohol.

Tinctures and ointments made from devil's claw were also very popular.

Warm baths and warm compresses were highly favored by those afflicted with lumbago.

## 73. CORNEA

As a preventive measure, it is advisable to thoroughly moisturize the body parts where calluses could form. For this purpose, udder ointment, marigold salve, and also deer tallow are suitable.

Dabbing with vinegar, especially apple cider vinegar, is a method to soften the calluses and make them easier to remove.

Also, applying warm, brewed chamomile to soften the calluses is an old home remedy. One can make a compress out of it or secure it with a bandage. After 20 to 40 minutes, the calluses should be nicely softened as a result.

Tying onion slices is also said to be helpful.

## 74. CORNS

Rub the affected area with garlic several times a day.

Rub the area with a piece of bacon rind from which the fat has been removed.

You can also use comfrey ointment. Apply it to the corns daily.

## COMFREY SALVE

Heat lard in a pan and add fresh, washed, and chopped comfrey roots. After it foams, stir and let the mixture cool overnight. Then warm it again to liquefy the mixture, pour it through a hair sieve or cloth, and squeeze the roots well. Fill the finished salve into small sealable jars and store them in a cool place.

Externally, a foot bath with boiled and strained nettle broth can also be helpful.

A cold infusion of nettles can also be used.

Nettle tea is preventive.

## NETTLE BROTH, COLD INFUSION

Put a few handfuls of nettles in several liters of cold water. Let it steep covered for about 8-12 hours. Afterwards, use this infusion with the nettles directly as a foot bath. To enhance its effectiveness, the infusion can also be .

Dabbing with nettle root tincture is also said to be helpful.

## NETTLE ROOT TINCTURE

> Fill a glass halfway with fresh, washed, and chopped nettle roots and pour spirits such as brandy or grain spirits over them. Let this sealed glass stand in a warm place for two weeks. Then strain, squeeze the roots well, and fill into brown bottles.

A plaster or cloth soaked with Swedish bitters and applied for several hours is also said to bring good results. If left on overnight, a sock can be worn over it to prevent soiling.

One can also tie a piece of pork rind, from which the fat has been removed, to the affected area or secure it with a plaster.

With a touch of magic, old folk medicine reads like this: Fix a small piece of bacon on the corn with a plaster, bury the bacon in the garden later; when it has rotted, the corn will also be gone, so they say.

Applying a plaster of grated onion and a little salt on the corn makes it soft and easy to remove after a few days.

## 75. COUGH, HOARNESS, MUMUGUOUS BRONCHIA

Horseradish juice mixed 1:1 with white wine vinegar, take 1 teaspoon every hour.

## HORSEREADISH JUICE

> Finely grate the horseradish, then thoroughly grind or crush with a mallet and extract the juice.

For coughs, honey mixed with dried peppermint herb was taken by the teaspoon.

Particularly in coastal regions, ingested herring milk was considered a remedy for coughs.

A tea made from woodruff herb was also said to be helpful.

Drink tea made from dried cherry stems. Stems from sour cherries are said to be particularly effective.

Barley tisane with honey was a folk medicine remedy.

In the southern region, it was common to smell crushed fresh ground-ivy - the smell alone was supposed to bring relief.

In Austria, a primrose tea was known as "Himmelbrand".

## COWSLIP FLOWER TEA

> 1 teaspoon of dried cowslip flowers are poured over with a cup of boiling water. Cover and let steep for 5 minutes, strain. The tea can also be sweetened with 1 tablespoon of honey.

Coltsfoot, collected in May as tea.

## COLTSFOOT TEA

1-2 tsp Coltsfoot leaves pour boiling water over with a cup of water, let it steep for 5 minutes. The tea should be taken for a maximum of 3 weeks.

Smoking Coltsfoot leaves or inhaling the smoke through a funnel is an old remedy for bronchitis. It is also said to be effective against smoker's cough.

A tea made from pine needles or pine tips helped to loosen mucus in cases of coughs and bronchitis.

Onion syrup is a folk remedy for coughs and hoarseness.

## ONION SYRUP

Peel and chop 1 onion, sprinkle with sugar in a glass. Take 2 tbsp of the resulting juice daily.

Taking a few drops of sunflower oil, about 1 hour after meals, is said to help with hoarseness.

Tea made from wood sanicle was a popular home remedy for coughs, lung problems, and catarrh.

## SANICLE TEA

> Pour 2 tsp of wood sanicle into a cup of boiling water, let it steep covered for 10 minutes, and strain. Drink 2 cups of it daily.

Honey without additives was already considered a remedy for coughs. Special effectiveness was attributed to forest honey.

Radish honey, take up to three times a day 2 tsp each.

## RADISH HONEY

> Hollow out radishes and fill the cavity with honey, place in a pot for about 6 hours. The liquid that forms is the radish honey.
>
> This cough syrup is particularly effective when made from black radish.

Radish juice with honey is also a home remedy for coughs and hoarseness. Take up to 3 times a day, 2 tsp each.

## RADISH JUICE WITH HONEY

> For radish juice with honey, grate the radishes finely, then mix with honey and let stand overnight. Then strain and squeeze out the radish pulp.

For coughs or as a preventive measure, you can chew licorice or drink licorice tea.

## LICORICE TEA

1-2 tsp grated licorice root

Pour 1 cup of boiling water over it, cover and let it steep for 15 minutes and strain. Drink the tea a maximum of 3 cups a day in small sips.

Pine needle honey is considered a mucus-loosening remedy for coughs.

## PINE NEEDLEHONEY

In spring, young spruce shoots are harvested. These are layered alternately with sugar in a glass. The layer of sugar should be about half the thickness of the shoots. Close the top layer with sugar and then let the glass stand closed on the windowsill until the contents have liquefied. Then strain the liquid and take it in teaspoonfuls.

Hot lemon is a proven remedy for coughs and hoarseness.

## HOT LEMON

> Squeeze the juice of 1/2 or one lemon without seeds
> into a glass. Add 1-2 tbsp of honey, fill with hot water,
> and stir. Drink as hot as possible in small sips.

Potato wraps are also said to help with persistent coughs.

## POTATO WRAP

> Cook 200 g of potatoes until tender, mash them finely,
> wrap in a cloth, flatten, place on the chest, and wrap
> with a cloth. Leave this wrap on for 30 minutes to an
> hour.

Ivy tea was an old remedy for coughs, especially when they were very persistent.

Marshmallow root syrup was used as a remedy for coughs, especially in children.

## MARSHMALLOW ROOT SYRUP

> Pour 100 g of marshmallow root, peeled, with 1.5 liters
> of hot water. Cover and let it stand for 10 minutes,
> then strain. Dissolve 1.5 kg of sugar in it. Then clarify
> the syrup with egg white. To do this, add the beaten
> egg whites of 2 eggs, wait until the foam has collected
> on the surface, and remove it by sieving. The syrup
> should be stored in a cool place. Take it by the
> teaspoonful as needed for coughs.

You can also prepare a cough tea that is widely used in folk medicine.

## COUGH TEA 1

- 4 tbsp of licorice root,
- 3 tbsp of fennel seeds
- 1 tbsp of anise seeds
- 2 2 tbsp of plantain leaves.

Mix well and add 1 teaspoon of boiling water if necessary. Leave covered for 10 minutes and strain. You can also sweeten the tea with a little honey.

## MARSHMALLOW TEA

Pour 1 tbsp of marshmallow herb with 1 cup of boiling water, cover for 10 minutes, and strain. Drink one cup in the morning and one in the evening.

## COUGH TEA 2

Boil 1 tbsp of plantain, 1 tbsp of thyme, and 1 tbsp of peppermint in 500 ml of water, let it steep for 10 minutes, and strain. You can sweeten the tea with a little honey.

## COUGH TEA 3

Pour the juice of 1/2 lemon over 3 tsp of anise, ground, and 3 tsp of thyme with 2 cups of boiling water, cover for 5 minutes, and drink as warm as possible.

Drink hot onion broth in sips.

## ONION BROTH

Peel an onion, cut it into pieces, and simmer in 1 liter of water for about 20 minutes. Then remove the onion and sweeten the broth with 3 tbsp of honey.

An onion tincture can also help, which is cooked longer than onion broth.

Peel and chop 2 onions, fry them in fat, and rub the neck, chest, and soles of the feet with the fat. Then put on a scarf and socks and go to bed to sweat.

Elecampane root, cooked in beer or honey, was already an effective remedy for coughs in the 17th century.

## ELECAMPANE HONEY

> Mix 1 tsp of ground elecampane root with 3 tbsp of
> honey. Take 1 tbsp three times a day.

Elecampane root was also used as a tea.

## ELECAMPANE ROOTTEA

> Pour 1 tsp of elecampane root with 1 cup of boiling
> water, cover for 15 minutes, and strain. Drink a cup
> three times a day.

Onion schnapps was also a remedy that was used. Take 1-2
tbsp three times a day.

## ONION SCHNAPPS

> Peel and chop onions. Put them in a glass and cover
> with brandy or fruit brandy until the onions are
> covered. Let it stand warm for a week.

Inhaling eucalyptus oil was recommended as helpful.

## EUCALYXPTUS INHALATION

> Boil 1 liter of water, let it cool slightly, add 3 drops of
> eucalyptus oil, hold your head over it as hot as
> possible, and cover your head and the pot with a cloth.

Birch bud tea is also a remedy for coughs.

BIRKENKNOSPEN-TEE

> 1 tbsp of birch buds, fresh Pour over with 2 cups of boiling water, let steep covered for 10 minutes, and drink one cup twice daily with a little honey.

Bitter larch bracket fungus (Laricifomes officinalis) was an old remedy for congested bronchi and lungs. For this, a knife tip of the powdered mushroom was taken.

## 76. HYPOCHONDRIA, ANXIETY, DEPRESSION

The biggest tip here is: Spend at least an hour exercising intensely outdoors daily.

Traveling with movement and physical as well as cultural activities lifts the mood and improves the outlook.

Horseback riding is a good balance and loosens tension, especially in the lower abdomen.

Dancing and outdoor games also help.

Warm and cold baths, including mineral baths, steam baths, and sweating baths, relax and refresh.

Drinking a cup of St. John's Wort tea daily or 1 tbsp of St. John's Wort tincture daily in tea or water were considered remedies to improve mood. However, it only takes effect when taken for a longer period of at least four weeks. St. John's Wort was also considered a good substitute for black tea.

### ST. JOHN'S WORT TEA

Pour 1-2 tsp of St. John's Wort with boiling water, cover for 10 minutes, and strain.

### ST. JOHN'S WORT TINCTURE

Fill a glass halfway with St. John's Wort flowers and leaves. Fill with at least 40% alcohol (vodka, grain alcohol), close, and let stand warm for 5-6 weeks. Shake daily. Then strain, pour the liquid into dark bottles, and close.

## 77. IMPOTENCE, STRENGTHENING MANHOOD

There are some foods recommended for increasing virility. These include asparagus, garlic, celery, eating eggs, and parsley.

## 78. INSECT STINGS

An old home remedy for bee stings is to crush the bee still on the sting site.

The sting should be removed with tweezers or fingertips.

Rubbing the bee sting with saliva or urine was an old home remedy used by farmers and forest workers.

Applying honey is also said to be very helpful, especially for bee stings.

For wasp stings or bee stings, it was recommended to apply a saltwater compress or freshly crushed parsley leaves or egg white or oil or honey, or wet soil, wet clay, wet loam, juice pressed from the stem of onions, juice from burdock leaves or sage leaves to the sting site.

Rubbing the sting site with a basil leaf was recommended.

Rubbing cow dung on the site is said to reduce itching and prevent swelling.

For ant bites, simply apply wet soil to the bite, it was recommended.

Rubbing mosquito bites with lemon juice.

For spider bites or stings, rub with oil.

For scorpion stings (perhaps they were only spiders), rub with oil or wash with vinegar and water.

It was also popular to crush or chew a plantain leaf and apply it to the sting.

You can also use a plantain tincture or a chamomile tincture by dabbing the insect sting with it.

## PLANTAIN TINCTURE

Fill a glass with plantain leaves and top it up with brandy or grain alcohol, making sure all leaves are well covered. Let this glass stand in a warm place for 5-6 weeks, shaking it daily if possible. Then strain and fill the liquid into brown bottles.

## CHAMOMILE TINCTURE

Fill a glass with chamomile flowers and top it up with brandy or grain alcohol, ensuring all flowers are well covered. Let this glass stand in a warm place for 5-6 weeks, shaking it daily if possible. Then strain and fill the liquid into brown bottles.

## CHAMOMILE TINCTURE, QUICK

Pour 5 tsp of chamomile with 200 ml of boiling water, let it steep for 10 minutes, strain, and press the liquid from the flowers. Once cooled, add 300 ml of brandy or grain alcohol to the obtained liquid. Fill the tincture into dark bottles if possible.

## 79. HANGOVER

The hangover after excessive drinking is not just a problem of modern times. Our ancestors also encountered the hangover and tried to combat it with home remedies.

To prevent the intoxication and subsequent hangover, ancient Romans used to eat several tablespoons of oil before drinking. Fatty and oily foods work very well here, such as oil sardines, especially when eaten without bread or other food.

A cold shower or bath was highly recommended.

A beer in the morning is said to chase away the hangover.

Some preferred chamomile tea to minimize the aftereffects, especially on the stomach.

Drinking a glass of water with a teaspoon of salt dissolved in it is said to dispel the hangover. The same is claimed for fizzy powder dissolved in water.

Spiced tomato juice, apple juice, and lemon juice were also popular remedies for the hangover.

Sour pickles, pickled cucumbers, vegetable or chicken soups, or a hearty meal were also popular remedies for the hangover, especially when accompanied by severe stomach discomfort.


## 80.  WHOOPING COUGH

To suppress the cough reflex, one should give mucilaginous drinks.

Rubbing onion juice into the soles of the feet is said to alleviate coughing.

Rubbing garlic juice mixed with lard on the back and stomach reduces coughing.

Strict diet should be observed.

The room should be well ventilated.

When the whooping cough is already beginning to subside, Icelandic moss was also used.

### ISLANDIC MOSS

The moss is soaked or boiled for 5-6 hours to remove impurities. Only then, take 1-2 tablespoons of moss per 1 liter of water and boil it down to 500 ml. Just before the end of boiling, add 1 tablespoon of licorice root or 1 tablespoon of anise and drink half a cup of it.

## 81. CHILDREN'S ISSUE

The best remedy for children and for preventing illness and strengthening health is to provide the child with good mother's milk for a long time.

In Bavaria 200 years ago, the following home remedy was common: Supplementing, nurturing: for weak mother's milk or prevented breastfeeding: offer diluted cow's milk boiled with some sugar from a nursing bottle. Offer semolina, white bread, or rice, cooked with milk or meat broth instead of milk, or give lukewarm whey or a mixture of 1/3 skimmed cow's milk with 3/4 oatmeal gruel.

If the baby is restless, it should be bathed in warm water and placed in bed with the mother.

For sore bottoms: apply baths of boiled bran and crushed carrots constantly.

If the eyelid is inflamed, a sponge was dipped in a strong infusion of elderberries and placed on the eyes.

Blackheads in children were coated with honey, then washed with soap.

For colic, anise tea or fennel tea was given. Massage the stomach with a warm hand during this time.

## ANISE TEA

Pour 1 teaspoon of crushed anise with boiling water, let it steep for 5 minutes, and strain.

If children wet the bed, they should be awakened once and taken to the toilet.

If there is foul-smelling discharge from the ears, a sponge was dipped in chamomile tea and pressed onto the ears. In addition, children were made to drink acorn coffee.

## ACORN COFFEE

Acorns are peeled and freed from the thin skin. To do this, briefly scald them with hot water or let them sit in cold water for 6 hours or longer until the skin can be removed. Then, the acorns are dried. To prepare acorn coffee, grind the dried acorns like regular coffee and steep 1 teaspoon of ground acorns with 1 cup of boiling water. Let it steep for 5 minutes and strain.

If the bowel movement of nursing children is delayed, they were given oatmeal gruel with honey.

"Dörrsucht" referred to the swelling of the abdomen in emaciation of the rest of the body, for which the breast of a healthy mother or wet nurse was given. If one was not available, cow's milk mixed with hearty beef soup was given.

For "English disease" (now rickets), much movement in fresh air was demanded as a home remedy, as well as cold and warm baths, meat, and acorn coffee were remedies against it.

To strengthen the children, cod liver oil was given for 3-4 weeks.

## 82. HEAD SCAB

To treat head scab, the hair was cut short.

The scab was loosened with warm linseed poultices, and then the head was repeatedly dabbed with sulfur water and rubbed with sulfur ointment in the evenings.

Alternatively, the bald head was also coated with olive oil and covered with crushed cabbage leaves. These were changed twice daily for 14 days.

## 83. HEAD SCAB, CRADLE CAP

If children have cradle cap, it should be treated by applying unsalted butter.

Sea baths or baths in saltwater (approximately 120 g of salt in 10 liters of water) were also believed to help alleviate cradle cap.

Washing with lukewarm water was thought to alleviate symptoms.

Applying an ointment made of fat and charcoal powder was also a common folk remedy. The charcoal powder was usually ground from softwoods.

Coating with olive oil and covering with white cabbage leaves were believed to soften and remove the scab.

Juniper berries were also crushed, boiled with a little water, and applied as a plaster together with lard.

## 84. HEAD LICE

Experience has shown that head lice were not only a problem in ancient times but have also reached modern times, particularly through contact in childcare facilities, and are again becoming prevalent.

Head lice were and are combed out with a nit comb. This procedure must be repeated as long as lice or nits are found.

Wine vinegar, diluted in a ratio of 100 ml of vinegar to 200 ml of water, used as a hair wash and left on for 10 minutes, supports treatment with the nit comb and should precede combing.

Applying an oil pack, whether olive oil or salad oil, left on for example for 2 hours to overnight, was believed to suffocate the lice.

Afterwards, the nits were combed out, and the hair was washed.

Essential oils such as eucalyptus, lavender, or rosemary were also used as home remedies against lice.

## HEAD LICE HAIR RINSE

- 5 drops of lavender oil
- 5 drops of rosemary oil
- 250 ml of white vinegar or apple cider vinegar
- 500 ml of water

Mix everything well and rinse the hair with it after washing. Without rinsing, wrap the head well and leave it on for 15 minutes. Then comb out with a nit comb, and finally, rinse the hair well again.

A decoction of bitterwood, massaged into the hair and left to dry, was also an effective remedy against head lice.

The quickest and most effective remedy was to completely and radically cut off the hair.

## 85. VARICOSE VEINS (DILATED BLOOD VEIN SWELLING)

In the past, varicose veins were rubbed with brandy or camphor, but also rubbed with poppy juice from unripe poppy capsules was common.

The varicose feet were wrapped with linen or flannel, or leather or dog fur stockings were used.

Diet was also considered a successful remedy.

Baths and showers with cold water were believed to help.

Compresses with mistletoe, which was formerly considered a witch's herb, were supposed to have a positive effect on varicose veins.

Compresses with a decoction of oak bark, horse chestnuts, or witch hazel are also very helpful.

Even a chestnut tea for internal use was recommended.

Good Henry was also placed on damp areas with the smooth side up and secured with a bandage.

Barefoot water walking in cold water is said to promote circulation and help with varicose veins.

Lemon peel in drinks strengthens the veins.

## 86. CRAMPS, MUSCLE CRAMPS

For cramps, the muscles were immediately tensed in the opposite direction of the cramp, i.e., pushed against the cramp.

For a calf cramp, the foot was gently pulled up with the leg extended.

Chamomile sitz baths were recommended for uterine cramps.

Some herbs were also used for cramps, including rosemary, basil, peppermint, lavender, and lemon balm.

Teas from these herbs can have preventive effects.

Milk and dairy products also prevent cramps, as do nuts, almonds, pine nuts, and sunflower seeds.

## 87. SCRATCHES AND ABRASIONS

Scratches and abrasions were cleaned with water and rubbed with lanolin, lard, or clarified butter.

## 88. GOITER

Lubrication with an iodine ointment was recommended for goiter.

The use of powdered sea sponge - **Euspongia officinalis - was** also **recommended**.

## 89. LIVER DISORDERS

For liver disorders, preparations such as tinctures and teas with milk thistle are said to help.

Also, taking 1 tablespoon of thistle oil in the morning and evening after meals, either ingested or dipped with bread, is said to be helpful.

Avoid any consumption of alcoholic beverages.

Artichoke juice and artichokes as vegetables are believed to strengthen the liver.

## 90. LUNG AILMENTS

Tea made from birch leaves is said to help with lung ailments.

Also, Linden ash (or the charcoal from it) in milk is believed to help. To prepare, mix a pinch of it in 1 glass of milk three times daily.

LINDEN CHARCOAL

> Use about 10 cm of the top branches of the lime tree
> and burn them so that only black charcoal remains.
> Grind this to a fine powder.

Even eggshells were used as a remedy for lung strength.

## EGGSHELL BRANDY

> Collect eggshells, dry them, and crush them. Then, soak
> them in brandy or grain alcohol and let the mixture sit for 3
> weeks in a warm place. Strain afterward. Drink 2-3 shot
> glasses of the solution daily.

## 91. STOMACH, UPSET

After overeating and thus having an upset stomach, drinking a glass of cold water slowly can be helpful.

Drinking artichoke juice or a decoction of artichoke, especially for pain caused by too much or too fatty food, can help.

Warm drinks like black coffee without milk and sugar or warm tea can help after meals.

The Romans used to drink hot water in such cases.

In France, it was common to drink sugar water.

Candied ginger or sugared calamus help with bloating and an overloaded stomach.

Some believe that drinking a glass of cherry brandy can also help with a full stomach.

Drinking pickle juice from salted or pickled cucumbers is also believed to help.

A salted herring or rollmop can relieve fullness.

A fully charred and ground cork from cork, mixed with water or milk and taken internally, can help.

Other finely ground charcoal from soft wood can also be used as a substitute for the charcoal tablets used today.

Taking a pinch of baking soda or baking powder dissolved in water can also help with stomach pain. The glass should be consumed quickly.

Peppermint oil is also used. Drip some peppermint oil onto a sugar cube and let it dissolve in the mouth.

An acorn coffee soothes the full stomach.

## ACORN COFFEE

Peel and skin the acorns. This is easier if you scald the acorns or let the peeled acorns soak in water for some time. Then, dry the acorns and grind them like coffee beans. For acorn coffee, use 1 teaspoon of acorn powder per 1 cup of boiling water and proceed as with the preparation of regular coffee.

All information and home remedies provided are for informational purposes only. They do not represent current scientific knowledge and are not intended for self-medication. Diagnosis and medication can only be carried out by a doctor or pharmacist.

## 92. STOMACHULCER, GASTRITIS

If you have stomach ulcers, you should not smoke, drink alcohol or coffee.

A white cabbage juice treatment over 2 weeks, where you drink around 300 ml of white cabbage juice throughout the day, should also help.

### WHITE CABBAGE JUICE

The white cabbage is finely grated, placed in a pot and salted well. Then mash vigorously with a paddle or similar until juice forms. Let it stand for several hours, then pour off the juice and squeeze out the white cabbage.

Linseed broth, taken 1 tablespoon in the morning and evening, but with an 8-day break, was also a folk medicine remedy.

### LINSEED BROTH

Soak 100 g of linseeds in 1 liter of water overnight, then strain. The liquid is then the linseed broth.

Chewing or consuming fennel or caraway seeds is always good for the stomach.

As light food, lightly salted oatmeal porridge or oatmeal soup, cooked with water, was recommended. A hearty chicken broth or chicken soup was also considered advisable light food.

Sugar and milk should be avoided.

Peppermint tea and other stomach teas should alleviate pain and soothe the stomach ulcer.

## STOMACH TEA

- 3 tbsp Lemon Balm Leaves
- 6 tbsp Peppermint Leaves
- 3 tbsp Chamomile Flowers
- 2 tbsp Anise Seeds

Pour 1 tbsp of the tea mixture with a cup of boiling water, let it steep covered for 10 minutes, and strain.

## 93. STOMACHCATARRH WITH FEVER

In the past an emetic was given.

Eating thin, slimy soups or water soups was a preferred method to cure the stomach.

Alcoholic beverages should not be consumed.

Only lukewarm water should be drunk.

## 94. STOMACH CRAMPS

For stomach cramps, especially when accompanied by bloating, drinking tea made from yarrow, peppermint, or fennel is recommended. Sodium carbonate was also taken.

In the south, especially in the Alps, musk yarrow (Achillea moschata) was highly valued. It acts like yarrow but is believed to be stronger. It was used as a tea but also processed into liqueurs and spirits.

### MUSK YARROW TEA

Pour 1 tsp of musk yarrow with a cup of boiling water and let it steep for 10 minutes. Then strain and drink hot. It can also be processed into mixed herbal tea with other herbs as desired.

It was also recommended to drink 1 tbsp of milk several times a day and rub warm oil on the stomach.

A sheet of blotting paper soaked in rum and placed on the stomach is said to help.

Others recommend eating or drinking several tablespoons of linseed oil.

Mixing 3-4 drops of cajeput oil with 1 tbsp of rum or spirit is said to alleviate acute cramps.

A home remedy that some might gladly follow: drinking 1 tsp of Madeira wine on an empty stomach in the morning for 8-14 days as a preventive measure and relief against stomach cramps.

Birch sap wine is also said to help against stomach cramps.

## BIRCH SAP WINE

3 tbsp fresh birch sap

1 cup white wine

Combine in a pot and warm without boiling. Then, drink in small sips.

Warm brandy compresses infused with crushed caraway seeds were applied to the stomach. Additionally, drinking marjoram tea was supportive.

## MAJORAM TEA

1 tsp dried marjoram
Steep in a cup of boiling water, covered, for 5 minutes. Then strain.

For stomach cramps, fennel tea, anise tea, or yarrow tea can be helpful.

## YARROW TEA

> 1-2 tsp dried yarrow herb and flowers Steep in a cup of boiling water, covered, for 5-10 minutes. Then strain.

In cases of stomach cramps associated with gallbladder issues, a mixture of linseed oil and sweet almond oil, with or without a little lemon juice, can be taken spoon by spoon throughout the day.

A tea made from avens, also known as wood avens or herb bennet (Geum urbanum), is not only considered a good substitute for black tea but also an excellent remedy for stomach cramps.

## AVENS TEA

> 1-2 tsp avens herb steeped in a cup of boiling water, covered, for 5-10 minutes. Then strain.

A tea made from blackthorn blossoms and fern was also considered a remedy for stomach cramps, as well as strong poppy seed tea, ginger tea, fennel tea, and Mexican tea (Dysphania ambrosioides), also known as Mexican wormseed.

# 95. STOMACH PAIN, ABDOMINAL PAIN

For abdominal and stomach pains, woolen abdominal wraps were worn to keep the stomach warm. Especially in children, a hot water bottle is also used.

Quark compresses were also considered helpful and recommended, along with consuming quark daily.

Cumin tea, peppermint tea, fennel tea, anise tea, chamomile tea, sage tea, and yarrow tea were popular teas used in such cases.

For children, fennel tea or chamomile tea is often the first choice.

## CUMIN TEA

To make cumin tea, add 1 teaspoon of cumin seeds to a cup and pour boiling water over them. Let it steep for 5-10 minutes, then strain.

## FENNEL TEA

For fennel tea, add 1 teaspoon of fennel seeds to a cup and pour boiling water over them. Let it steep for 10 minutes, then strain.

Onion tincture was not only a remedy for coughs but also for stomach pains.

## ONION TINCTURE

- 500 ml water
- 250 g onions
- 200 g sugar
- 25 g honey

> Peel and chop the onions. Then simmer them with water and honey in a pot for at least 1 hour. Strain the liquid, squeeze out the onions, and pour the hot liquid into a bottle and seal tightly. Larger quantities can be made, but after opening the bottles, the tincture should be refrigerated and consumed within approximately 2-3 days.

Chewing cumin seeds is said to help with stomach pains.

A tried-and-true remedy for stomach pains is a hot water bottle, a hot stone, or a warm cherry stone pillow placed on the stomach under the covers.

It was recommended to slightly bend the legs, as this helps alleviate the pain more quickly.

A linen pouch filled with oats and placed on the stomach was also used.

The oats should be lightly moistened, warmed, and placed in the pouch.

Taking up to 20 drops of elecampane tincture up to 3 times a day is said to help the stomach.

Tea made from sloe flowers, elderflowers, or peppermint is said to help with stomach pains.

SLOE FLOWER TEA Collect and dry the flowers. To make tea, pour 1 teaspoon of the flowers into a cup of boiling water and let it steep for 5 minutes. Ginger is also a remedy that was used for stomach pains. GINGER TEA Thinly peel and grate a piece of ginger about half the length of your thumb. Then pour boiling water over it, let it steep for 10 minutes, and strain. Sauerkraut was eaten or its juice was drunk for stomach pains. Freshly grated white cabbage or red cabbage juice was also believed to be helpful. True Curacao bitter liqueur with an addition of bishop's extract was considered one of the best remedies for stomach issues. Bitter larch fungus - Laricifomes officinalis - was a proven remedy for stomach pains.

## SLOE FLOWER TEA

Collect and dry the flowers. To make tea, pour 1 teaspoon of the flowers into a cup of boiling water and let it steep for 5 minutes

Ginger is also a remedy that was used for stomach pains.

## GINGER TEA

Thinly peel and grate a piece of ginger about half the length of your thumb. Then pour boiling water over it, let it steep for 10 minutes, and strain.

Sauerkraut was eaten or its juice was drunk for stomach pains.

Freshly grated white cabbage or red cabbage juice was also believed to be helpful.

True Curacao bitter liqueur with an addition of bishop's extract was considered one of the best remedies for stomach issues.

Bitter larch fungus - Laricifomes officinalis - was a proven remedy for stomach pains.

## LARCH SPONGE MILK

Boil 1 tablespoon of chopped or ground fungus in 500 ml of milk, and simmer for almost 30 minutes. Then strain and drink.

## 96. TONSILLITIS

Dissolving honey cake in hot goat's milk and drinking it teaspoon by teaspoon was believed to help. This home remedy was widely practiced in southern Germany, particularly in Bavaria.

For suppurating tonsils, inducing vomiting by inserting a feather dipped in oil into the throat to encourage the abscess to burst was done.

Cooling compresses around the neck were also a preferred method. Quark compresses, where the quark is applied to the neck, are an old home remedy. Variations of these wraps included a mixture of quark and vinegar.

Wraps with potatoes cooked as jacket potatoes, which are placed hot in a cloth and applied to the neck or chest, were also believed to help.

Steam baths with sage or chamomile and inhaling the hot vapors were thought to provide relief.

## 97. MEASLES

Strict bed rest in a slightly darkened, quiet room was customary during measles.

Drinking plenty of fluids was also recommended.

For high fever, calf compresses with a mixture of water and vinegar were used.

As for food, light meals, especially the popular chicken soup of the time, were served.

## 98. MENSTRUAL PROBLEMS

Chamomile tea can be helpful for menstrual cramps.

Tea made from lemon balm is also believed to help.

For menstrual problems, lady's mantle tea was recommended.

It is consumed daily, 2-3 cups, from one week before menstruation until the end of menstruation. It is advisable to check for any symptoms after a few months.

## LADY'S MANTLE TEA

> The tea can be made from dried or fresh herb. Brew 2 teaspoons of fresh lady's mantle herb or 1 teaspoon of dried lady's mantle herb with a cup of boiling water, let it steep for 10 minutes, and strain.

There were also blends of lady's mantle tea with dead nettle, lemon balm, or chamomile. In this case, use 2 teaspoons of lady's mantle and 1 teaspoon of the other herb.

Lady's mantle dew can also be collected, which is believed to have similar effects.

## LADY'S MANTLE DEW

> In the morning, you can collect the dew that has settled on the leaves of lady's mantle with a pipette, which the plant sweats or secretes.

# 99. MIGRAINE, HEADACHES

Rubbing sea salt with egg white and applying it to the forehead and temples while keeping the feet warm was believed to help.

It was also recommended to drink a cup of strong coffee or green tea. To enhance the effect, lemon can be added to the coffee.

Snuffing tobacco was also believed to be helpful.

Some people also applied lemon peel to their temples. The lemon peel was cut into a round shape with a diameter of about 2 cm, all the white parts were removed, and then it was attached to the temple with the moist side, causing a red spot to appear, which was believed to relieve the migraine.

In Italy, peach leaves were tied to the forehead. Similarly, a fresh cabbage leaf bound to the forehead was believed to help.

Another home remedy involved dipping a piece of bread crust in vinegar and binding it to the forehead.

Warming vinegar and mixing it with soap to wash the forehead and temples was also believed to be helpful.

A foot bath with 5 liters of warm water and 15 g of mustard flour added was believed to be beneficial for headaches.

Drinking a tea made from crushed juniper berries was also believed to help.

Massaging the temples with lavender oil, peppermint oil, or rubbing alcohol was also a home remedy.

The simplest home remedy was to lie in bed in a dark, quiet room and wait for the headaches to subside.

## 100.　　MUSCLE SORENESS,STRAINS

It was recommended to wear warming bandages. Bandages were also used when joints were affected.

Massaging the sore areas thoroughly with olive oil or lanolin was beneficial.

Marigold or arnica, as ointments, tinctures for rubbing, or compresses made from the herbs or tea, were also considered helpful.

Rubbing alcohol was commonly used in earlier times. It can be rubbed onto the affected areas.

For strains and sprains, compresses made from a paste of fresh comfrey or alant leaves or a decoction of the leaves were applied.

## 101.　　BIRTHMARK

To lighten the appearance of a birthmark, the heart or core was extracted from the borage root, which forms a white streak in the middle. This was soaked in wine vinegar, and then the liquid was repeatedly applied to the spots with a sponge.

## 102.     UMBILICAL HERNIA

A very old home remedy was to attach 1/2 nutmeg or a walnut of appropriate size with large adhesive tape to the navel. This was done to push back the intestine protruding through the hernia and hope for the hernia to heal again. This home remedy was particularly used for children.

## 103.     NAIL FUNGUS

Moistening or spraying with vinegar was a simple home remedy for stubborn nail fungus. In more recent times, apple cider vinegar has been commonly used.

Keeping the feet dry is important.

## 104.     NOSEBLEEDS

A simple remedy to stop the flow of blood from the nose is to lean forward while simultaneously pinching the nostrils shut with the hand for about 5-10 minutes.

Forming a plug from cotton and tinder fungus, dipping it in vinegar, and then plugging the bleeding nostril with it was a popular home remedy.

Some people also inserted a piece of bacon into the nostril.

Alternatively, small cloths soaked in lemon juice were inserted into the nostrils.

Birch fungus was burned, powdered, and sniffed.

Rinsing the nose with water or water mixed with a little vinegar was a folk remedy to stop nosebleeds.

Applying cold compresses to the neck or genital area was believed to stop the flow of blood, as well as taking cold foot baths.

Applying a cold compress with cold water, or if available, with ice cubes wrapped in a cloth, to the bridge of the nose or the neck was also believed to be helpful.

One could also soak a cloth or compress in witch hazel tea or witch hazel tincture and hold it on or in the nostril.

It was also recommended to place a halved onion or a cold cloth on the back of the neck to stop nosebleeds.

## 105.     HIVES

For hives, elderberry tea or elderflower tea was traditionally consumed.

Avoiding meat was also recommended.

## 106.        TINNITUS

For tinnitus, people felt compelled to clean their ears with an ear spoon.

Cotton was also inserted into the outer ear and moistened with garlic juice or onion juice.

Foot baths with ash were also believed to help.

## 107.        EARACHE

Crush a leaf of cranesbill (also known as herb robert or storksbill) and insert it into the ear.

Crush a geranium leaf and insert it into the ear.

Lightly crush a garlic clove and insert it into the ear. It was also wrapped in a cloth before being inserted into the ear. It was common to squeeze the clove onto a cloth until it was soaked with juice, then place it in or on the ear.

You can also make a poultice with onion. Chop a small onion, wrap it in a cloth, and place it behind the painful ear. In the past, onion pieces were often inserted into the ear or an onion slice was tied onto the ear.

A more modern method is to extract juice from onion or garlic and put a few drops of the juice into the ear. It is advisable to seal the ear with cotton or similar afterward.

Allowing steam to enter the ear was also practiced.

Applying 1-2 drops of warmed oil, such as olive oil, may help with earaches. Chamomile oil was also used; it could be made by mixing 3 tbsp of olive oil or sunflower oil with 1 tbsp of chamomile flowers and letting it stand in a small glass jar sealed overnight.

Before the invention of electricity, the ear was kept warm with a hot water bottle, or by sitting near a warm oven with the ear facing it. After the invention of electricity, this function was taken over by the heat lamp.

Applying poultices of mustard flour, left on for about 10 minutes once a day, was believed to be helpful.

You can also apply poultices made from flaxseed or chamomile. Fenugreek may also help.

Allowing vapors from hot elderberry tea or elderflower tea to enter the ear was also a remedy for earaches.

## ELDERBERRY TEA

Steep 1 teaspoon of dried elderberries in 1 cup of boiling water. Let it steep for 5 minutes, then strain.

> Steep 2 teaspoons of elderflowers in 1 cup of boiling
> water. Let it steep for 10 minutes, then strain.

Drip a few drops of sweet almond oil or lukewarm milk into the ear daily.

Additionally, herbal teas were administered for support, such as teas made from lime blossoms, burdock root, peppermint, mullein, elderflower, or angelica root, either individually or mixed.

## 108.     FACIAL PIMPLES, ACNE

In the morning before eating, pimples were dabbed with fresh saliva or fresh urine. This remedy is particularly suitable for inflamed pimples.

Washing the face with bran should cleanse the skin.

Treatment with chamomile tincture or arnica tincture was also believed to be promising.

Dabbing the pimples with a cut garlic clove was also believed to help with pimples.

Dabbing with wine vinegar or apple cider vinegar also helps to open up the pores and make the pimple disappear.

Steam baths with chamomile are also helpful.

Tea tree oil, dabbed on, is said to dry out pimples.

An old remedy was also classic zinc ointment, which was supposed to dry out pimples.

## 109.　　BRUISES

Bruises - they happen quickly with heavy work and also with activities outdoors. But even in the household, one can bruise easily.

First and foremost, cooling was usually applied. This involved compresses with cloths soaked in cold water or even wrapped ice packs.

Another "quick fix" was to moisten the bruise with one's own urine.

Since it's always readily available, it was the fastest self-help one could administer.

Also, rubbing with the formerly widely used rubbing alcohol (in german: Franzbranntwein) was common.

A popular remedy in the past was a compress with boiled and mashed potatoes. These were wrapped in a cloth and applied as hot as possible to the bruise.

Compresses with quark were also believed to be helpful.

Additionally, bruises were smeared with clay or mud - nowadays, vinegar compound clay is surely used.

But compresses with arnica flowers, marjoram herb, parsley, or comfrey roots were also common.

## ARNICA FLOWER COMPRESS

Infuse 3 tablespoons of arnica flowers in 2 cups of boiling water. Let it steep for 10 minutes. Then, strain the liquid, or directly soak a cloth in it and apply it to the bruise.

## MAJORAM COMPRESS

Crush several marjoram leaves, mix them with some honey, and apply to the affected area. Alternatively, you can directly apply the crushed marjoram leaves to the bruise.

## PARSLEY COMPRESS

Finely chop parsley, mix it with an egg white, and spread the mixture onto a cloth. Place this on the painful area.

Bruises were also treated with arnica ointment.

Cold compresses were applied for cooling. This was done with cold water or ice cubes wrapped in a cloth.

Here, a compress with vinegar or apple cider vinegar was recommended for about 1 minute, then rubbed with Arnica tincture.

The Arnica tincture was also applied as a compress, meaning a cloth was moistened with the Arnica tincture and placed on the affected area. This was repeated when the cloth dried out.

## ARNICA TINCTURE – OLD METHOD

Arnica herb (root, herb, flower) is collected during springtime when it blooms, crushed, and the juice is extracted. Then, the juice is mixed with an equal amount of high-proof alcohol. The resulting light-colored liquid is the Arnica tincture. However, the tincture is so potent that before use, it is diluted by mixing 100 drops with 250 ml of water. This mixture is then ready for use.

## ARNICA TINCTURE

Fill a glass halfway with Arnica herb, then fill it with brandy until the herbs are well covered. Let the tincture stand for 6 weeks in a warm place, shaking it occasionally. Then, filter the tincture and pour it into a dark bottle. It is best to store the tincture in a cool, dark place. The tincture lasts at least 1 year.

Compresses with wine or brandy were also common remedies.

Compresses made from lemon balm leaves and rye bread were also used.

## LEMON BALM BREAD COMPRESS

> Lemon balm leaves and bread are mixed with a little vinegar to create a thick paste. This paste is applied to the affected area and covered.

For severe bruises with bruised areas, leeches were applied to the affected area.

## 110.     PROSTATE PROBLEMS

Prostate issues were particularly common among older men.

Sitz baths with horsetail infusion were considered helpful.

As preventive measures and aids, teas made from nettle root or willowherb were consumed.

## NETTLE ROOT TEA

> Boil 1 tablespoon of dried nettle root in a pot with one
> cup of water for 2 minutes. Then, let it steep covered
> for 10 minutes, and strain. Drink up to three cups of
> this tea daily.

## WILLOWHERB TEA

> Pour 1 teaspoon of willowherb into a cup of boiling
> water. Let it steep for 10 minutes, then strain. Drink
> one cup in the morning and one in the evening.

## 111.  MENSTRUAL CYCLE, IRREGULAR

Drinking wormwood tea regularly is believed to help regulate the menstrual cycle.

## WORMWOOD TEA

> Pour 1 teaspoon of wormwood into a cup of boiling
> water and let it steep covered for 10 minutes. Then
> strain. This bitter tea can also be sweetened with some
> honey.

Mugwort has been used since the 16th century as a remedy for irregular menstrual cycles. It was used as a tea or tincture.

## MUGWORT TEA

> Pour 1-2 teaspoons of mugwort herb into a cup of boiling water and let it steep covered for 10 minutes. Then strain. This tea can also be sweetened with some honey.

One of the oldest recipes is mugwort wine.

## MUGWORT WINE

> Boil a handful of mugwort herb in 600 ml of white wine until it reduces to 1/3, then drink a cupful in the morning and evening.

## 112. MENSTRUAL FLOW, TOO LIGHT

A tea made from yarrow was recommended to help with light menstrual flow.

## 113. MENSTRUAL FLOW, TOO HEAVY

For heavy menstrual flow, drinking oak bark tea in small sips was recommended.

## OAK BARK TEA

> Steep 1 teaspoon of dried, crushed oak bark in a cup
> of boiling water, cover and let it steep for 15 minutes,
> then strain.

Mistletoe tea was also recommended for excessive bleeding.

## 114.     RHEUMATISM

For rheumatism without fever, rubbing with cologne water, rum, or brandy was recommended. The limb was then wrapped in linen, waxed linen, or tanned rabbit or hare skin. Also common was the application of fresh wool from sheep's fleece or wrapping with wool or cotton that had been smoked with the fumes of sugar, amber, juniper, or mastic.

An old home remedy was to bury a piece of linen in an anthill overnight, which was then used to wrap the rheumatic limb.

In regions where wine was produced, the grape press residues were also commonly used as a rheumatism compress.

Relief was also thought to come from crusts of still warm fresh bread, which were applied. Overall, many methods aimed to alleviate rheumatic pains with heat or cold.

Steam baths, sauna, and hot mud or mud baths can be helpful as long as the symptoms are not accompanied by fever.

The painful areas were also rubbed with rosemary tincture.

Rubbing alcohol was used for rubbing. Sometimes a pine rubbing alcohol tincture was also used for rubbing.

## PINE RUBBING ALCOHOL TINCTURE

A sealable glass is filled halfway with spruce shoots and topped up with rubbing alcohol (in german: Franzbranntwein) so that the shoots are well covered. Then, it is left closed in a warm place for 2-3 weeks, shaking it daily. Afterward, it is strained, poured into dark bottles, and sealed. This tincture was used exclusively for rubbing and massaging for rheumatism and gout.

St. John's Wort oil was also used for rubbing in cases of rheumatism.

## ST. JOHN'S WORT OIL

A sealable glass is filled halfway with St. John's Wort and topped up with olive oil, ensuring everything is well covered. Then, it is left closed in a warm place for 5-6 weeks, shaking it daily. Afterward, it is strained, poured into dark bottles, and sealed.

Sulfur baths were recommended for rheumatism and gout. The affected body parts were bathed in the solution.

Milk baths, that is, warm baths with the addition of milk, were especially recommended for older people.

Baths with warm water infused with mistletoe tea were also said to help against rheumatism.

## SULFUR BATH

30 g of sulfur liver and 60 g of soap are boiled in 5 liters of water.

Common restharrow tea is said to be helpful against rheumatism. You drink up to 2 cups daily spread throughout the day.

## COMMON RESTHARROW TEA

Steep 2 teaspoons of common restharrow herb and root in 250 ml of water, let it sit for 10 minutes, then strain.

The fresh plant juice of the artichoke is also said to have a positive effect on rheumatism and gout. To use, take one teaspoon of the juice every 2 hours, mixed with honey or sugar syrup.

Rheumatism teas were also commonly used.

## RHEUMATISM TEA

3 tablespoons of celery leaves
2 tablespoons of common restharrow
2 tablespoons of peppermint herb
1 tablespoon of calamus
1 tablespoon of rose hips

> 1 tablespoon of chamomile flowers
> Mix everything well, brew 1 teaspoon of the mixture
> with a cup of boiling water, let it steep for 5 minutes,
> strain, and drink 1 cup daily in the morning and
> evening.

## 115.      RUBELLA (GERMAN MEASLES)

For rubella, bed rest was observed.

It was also recommended to drink plenty of fluids. In case of high fever, cold calf compresses with a water-vinegar mixture were applied.

Quark compresses helped relieve itching.

## 116.      BACK PAIN

The simplest home remedy for back pain is a warm bath.

Intensively massaging oil or ointment onto the affected areas provides relief.

Recommended oils include pine oil, ginger oil, or sandalwood oil.

If you have nothing else at home, you can use olive oil and massage it into the affected areas.

Also, rubbing with tinctures of ash, oak bark, and poplar can be helpful.

 A warming and helpful effect can be achieved with chili extract.

Salves based on marigold or devil's claw are also said to be helpful.

For lumbago, it was recommended to cover the back with flannel and iron it with a warm iron.

## 117.    SCARLETFEVER

For scarlet fever accompanied by fever, bed rest was advised.

It was also important to drink plenty of fluids.

Cold calf compresses with a water-vinegar mixture were applied in case of high fever.

To alleviate sore throat, gargling with diluted watered-down wine vinegar or apple cider vinegar was recommended. Some also added 1 tablespoon of honey to this water.

## 118.    VAGINITIS

A tried and tested remedy here is a sitz bath with chamomile.

## 119.    VAGINAL YEAST INFECTION

One recommendation was to wear quark compresses in underwear or insert quark directly.

## 120.    BURSITIS, TENDINITIS

One should avoid excessive movement; if that's not possible, a bandage could help.

Quark compresses were very helpful in relieving symptoms.

Here, too, the obligatory quark compresses or compresses with crushed cabbage leaves were applied.

A linseed poultice could also help.

### FLAXSEED POULTICE

Flaxseeds are boiled in a small amount of water. The resulting paste is spread on a linen or cotton cloth, placed on the affected area, and tied firmly with another cloth or bandage.

## 121.        SWALLOWING, CHOKIN

The simplest tip is to hold your breath for some time.

A recommendation sometimes followed was to drink a small glass of rum in small sips.

Drinking cold water in tiny sips without breathing is also said to help.

Others suggested drinking a bit of lemon juice or vinegar.

Further recommendations included drinking several cups of chamomile tea or spearmint tea.

### SPEARMINT TEA

1 teaspoon dried spearmint
 Pour boiling water over the peppermint in 1 cup, let steep covered for 5 minutes.

Inducing sneezing by letting the sun shine on the nose or tickling the nose could also be helpful.

## 122.        CUTS

For knife cuts on the finger, dip them in salt or paprika powder or cayenne pepper.

To stop the bleeding: Dip cotton wool in hot water and press it on the wound.

Small cuts on the fingers or hands were treated with one's own urine. (easy for men - just pee on it)

Applying freshly ground chamomile herb is also said to promote healing. The cut was treated with preferably still warm arnica-pine ointment.

## ARNICA-PINE OINTMENT

Heat 2 tablespoons of butter with 3 crushed arnica flowers, a hazelnut-sized piece of pine resin or spruce resin, and some chamomile flowers, stirring well.

Cuts were also treated with pine resin ointment.

## PINE RESIN OINTMENT

Put pine resin in a pot and bring to a boil. Discard the liquid, and mix the sediment with oil in a ratio of 1:3.

Making a compress with sauerkraut juice is also said to have helped. A linen cloth was dipped in sauerkraut juice and bound to the wound. This was changed several times.

## 123.     COMMON COLD

An old remedy for a cold is to blow your nose thoroughly and breathe deeply through the nose.

In France, a glass of hot sugar water mixed with an egg yolk was consumed.

A chamomile steam bath was also very helpful. This was applied up to 3 times daily.

## CHAMOMILE STEAM BATH

> Infuse 3 teaspoons of chamomile in a pot with 500 ml of boiling water. Lean your head over the pot and cover both your head and the pot with a towel. Breathe predominantly through your nose. You can also add some Arnica tincture to the water.

For a congested nose, a steam bath of hot water and wine vinegar should be made.

Rinsing the mouth and nose with elderflower water should also help.

## ELDERFLOWER WATER FOR RINSING

> Add 2-3 handfuls of dried elderflowers to 1 liter of water, bring to a boil, let it steep for a while, strain, and add a splash of vinegar to the water.

Drinking fennel tea is not only a good remedy for the stomach but also for a stuffy nose.

## FENNEL TEA

> Put 1-2 teaspoons of fennel seeds in a cup and pour boiling water over them. Let it steep covered for 5 minutes, then strain.

Drinking coltsfoot tea with honey is a remedy deeply rooted in folk medicine for centuries, effective against colds, coughs, and more.

## COLTSFOOT TEA

> Infuse 1-2 teaspoons of finely chopped and dried coltsfoot leaves with a cup of boiling water, let it steep for 5 minutes, then strain. You can sweeten the tea with honey.
>
> For a cough tea, you can also combine coltsfoot with licorice root, anise seeds, marshmallow root, and coltsfoot flowers.

## 124.  DANDRUFF, SCALPY SCALP

One remedy used was to wash the head with nettle tea and massage it well into the scalp.

Also, a mixture consisting of 1 tablespoon of almond oil and 3 drops of rosemary oil, massaged in after shampooing, was said to eliminate dandruff.

Wine vinegar or fruit vinegar was used against dandruff. It was massaged into the scalp without rinsing out. Sometimes nettle leaves, lavender, rosemary, or willow bark were steeped in boiling vinegar and this solution was used.

Rinses of birch water, chamomile tea, or nettle tea were believed to eliminate dandruff. Also, massaging with tea tree oil or burdock seed oil has proven effective.

Another home remedy is to whisk 2 egg yolks and massage them into the scalp. Leave this on for 15 minutes and then rinse with beer.

A mixture of lemon juice and egg yolk, applied before washing and allowed to sit briefly, is also said to help with dandruff.

A hair tonic made from a brew of nettle leaves boiled in fruit vinegar or wine vinegar is believed to be helpful against dandruff.

Washing with a brew of maidenhair fern or venus hair (Adiantum capillus-veneris) should also help with dandruff.

## MAIDENHAIR FERN HAIR WASH

2-4 tablespoons of maidenhair fern boiled in 500 ml of water, steeped for 10 minutes, strained, and the solution massaged into the hair and scalp.

## 125.        SWEATING, EXCESSIVE

If one suffered from excessive foot sweating, it was recommended to sprinkle fresh wheat bran into the socks daily and wear them, but to avoid woolen socks. Also, washing the feet in the morning with rubbing alcohol or pouring some into shoes or boots was an old folk remedy.

For excessive hand sweating, rubbing the hands with rubbing alcohol was recommended.

Sage tea, mixed with red wine, was supposed to reduce excessive body sweat. Also, drinking English porter or two glasses of donkey milk mixed with a tablespoon of rum daily, or rubbing the affected areas with olive oil every 3-4 days, was said to help.

Baths with chamomile for affected hands or feet were said to provide relief.

## 126.        SEASICKNESS, TRAVEL SICKNESS

For seasickness, ginger was the remedy of choice. It was chewed as a whole piece, drunk as ginger tea, or consumed as ginger liqueur.

## 127.        HEARTBURN

Against heartburn, one can peel and chew or eat 2 fresh acorns, or eat 2 dried and ground acorns.

A small glass of gentian schnapps is said to help against heartburn and was widely used as folk medicine in southern Germany.

Against morning heartburn, drinking a glass of sugar water may help.

Mixing 1 teaspoon of baking soda or bicarbonate of soda in a glass of water and drinking it can help. Magnesia or chalk powder can also be used.

An old remedy was also the use of effervescent powder. This was either mixed in a glass and drunk with water or taken directly into the mouth and water drunk afterward.

## EFFERVESCENT POWDER

3 tablespoons of baking soda
2 tablespoons tartaric acid
2 tablespoons of sugar

Everything was mixed and stored dry until use. A normal dose is 1-2 teaspoons.

A very old remedy for heartburn is also the intake of roasted and ground eggshells. About 1-1.5 grams of these were taken in water.

Dry zwieback, baked without yeast, is an old remedy for gastric acid. Old, dry bread also served this purpose.

## 128.　　　SUNBURN

Quark compresses help and soothe sunburn.

Clay compresses were also made for severe sunburn.

## 129.　　　STONES, GRAVEL, BLADDER STONES, KIDNEY STONES

Over time, acidic foods such as sauerkraut, lemon, dishes with vinegar, etc., were supposed to reduce and expel the stones or dissolve gravel in the bladder or kidney.

Birch water was also considered a diuretic, as were almost all diuretic herbs and plants.

The same was hoped for when using birch leaves, birch bark, nettles, goldenrod, butcher's broom, couch grass, and lovage. The herbs and plants are mostly diuretic and were supposed to flush out the stones. The teas were used 3-4 times a day.

### GOLDENROD TEA

Steep 1-2 teaspoons of goldenrod herb in 1 cup of boiling water, cover and let it infuse for 10 minutes, then strain.

## LOVAGE TEA

Brew 1 teaspoon of lovage with 1 cup of boiling water, cover, let it steep for 5 minutes, then strain.

## COUCH GRASS ROOT TEA

Infuse 2 teaspoons of chopped couch grass root, fresh or dried, in 1 cup of boiling water, cover, let it steep for 15 minutes, then strain and drink.

## BUTCHER'S BROOM TEA

Steep 1 teaspoon of dried butcher's broom root in 1 cup of boiling water, cover, let it infuse for 10 minutes, then strain.

Marshmallow was also a home remedy for urinary tract issues.

## MARSHMALLOW TEA

Boil 1 tablespoon of marshmallow leaves or roots in a pot with 250 ml of water for about 3 minutes. Then strain and drink 2 cups per day.

Here's an old recipe for a tea against stones and gravel.

> 2 tablespoons of birch leaves
> 2 tablespoons of couch grass
> 2 tablespoons of speedwell
> 2 tablespoons of chicory
>
> Infuse 1 teaspoon of each with a cup of boiling water, let it steep for 10 minutes, and drink a cup 3 times a day.

## 130. RESTLESS SLEEP, BAD DREAMS

Sleeping with the head elevated should help against bad dreams and restless sleep.

Drinking a glass of sugar water in the evening should also be helpful.

Avoiding meat in the diet should lead to a peaceful sleep.

It was recommended to particularly avoid meat in the evening.

## 131. BURNS, MINOR

In folk medicine, burns were dusted with flour and bandaged, then after some time, the burnt skin was cleaned with arnica tincture.

Applying honey is said to prevent blistering and scarring from burns or scalds.

Burns were often treated with a mixture of olive oil and egg white.

Closed burn wounds were rubbed with a halved onion.

Witch hazel ointment, witch hazel oil, and witch hazel tincture were home remedies for treating burns.

Also, compresses of cloths soaked in witch hazel tea were applied.

In Mecklenburg, it was common to treat burns with a butter ointment.

## BUTTER OINTMENT

40 g Unsalted Butter
20 g Mutton Tallow
20 g Beeswax

The ointment is melted together and thoroughly mixed. Then, it is poured into small jars and sealed.

## 132.	CONSTIPATION

Eating one or two apples or drinking apple juice can already help.

A simple remedy was fresh sauerkraut for breakfast or taking 1-2 tablespoons of oil.

Olive oil or linseed oil was recommended as the oil, if it doesn't work, repeat after a few hours. If none of these work, enemas were administered. Warm water or a mixture of water and milk was used for this purpose. Sometimes, oil was also added.

Soaking 6 dried plums and 6 dried figs in a little water for 15 hours, eating the fruit before bedtime, and drinking the water the next day in sips, was recommended by our ancestors for those suffering from constipation.

Suppositories made from soap are also an old-time remedy.

Taking a hazelnut-sized piece of soap up to 3 times is said to have a similar effect.

Eating dried plums is said to get digestion back on track and relieve constipation.

Especially in Italy and France, cooked tomatoes were recommended as a remedy for constipation.

Cherries, grapes, blackberries, etc., are said to ensure regular bowel movements.

Milk, buttermilk, baked apples, cooked plums, red cabbage, kale, and sauerkraut are also said to ensure a regular passage.

As a spring cure for digestion, the herbs of dandelion, cumin, chervil, sorrel, and chicory, cooked like spinach, were eaten.

Sour apples, fried or braised in olive oil, along with a cup of hot milk or coffee, are also said to help.

Fresh grape, pear, or apple juice is also said to be highly effective.

Senna leaves (Alexandrian Senna - Senna alexandrina) and rhubarb (leaves, root, cooked) have a laxative effect. The following tea was also used as a laxative.

## LAXATIVE TEA

1 teaspoon of chamomile flowers is steeped in a cup of boiling water. Let it sit covered for 5 minutes, then stir in 1 teaspoon of honey and 1 teaspoon of flaxseed oil. Drink 2-3 cups of this tea daily until you notice results.

For children, raisins dipped in oil or small, elongated bars of soap were administered as suppositories to induce bowel movements.

Another remedy for children was a cup of rhubarb juice mixed with 1 tablespoon of honey.

Tea made from peach blossoms and wild rose petals was also believed to have a laxative effect.

Elm leaves, soaked cold in water for several hours, were a proven remedy for constipation.

Another remedy involved milk with honey and brewer's yeast.

For women suffering from chronic constipation, it was advised to consume 2-3 teaspoons of Epsom salt (magnesium sulfate) in unsalted broth.

For elderly individuals, a laxative recommended was coffee with senna leaves. 4-5 grams of senna leaves were added to a cup of coffee.

Castor oil was also used for its laxative properties.

## 133.    WARTS

In the past, warts were often healed through rituals, incantations, and "prayer."

Letting live black slugs crawl over the wart was believed to make it fall off.

Simply crushing fresh black currants on the warts.

Applying the yellow-orange juice from celandine several times a day is said to make warts disappear.

Rubbing the wart with a so-called "devil's stone pencil" (silver nitrate) burns it and causes it to fall off.

Dabbing the wart with castor oil 2-3 times daily for 2-3 weeks.

It is also believed to be helpful to place a slice of garlic on the wart and leave it on with a plaster for about a week.

Brushing the wart with thuja tincture.

Dropping lemon juice onto the wart is also said to help.

## TREEOF LIVE TINCTURE AGAINST WARTS

- 40 g fresh arborvitae twigs, chopped
- 60 ml alcohol, preferably 68-70%

Place the twigs in a glass, pour the alcohol over them, seal the glass, and let it sit in a warm place, such as by the window, for about 3 weeks, shaking daily. Then strain through a sieve, squeeze out the twigs, and store in a dark bottle.

Alternatively, high-proof vodka can be used.

This tincture is ONLY for warts. Note: Arborvitae is toxic and can also trigger allergies.

Fig warts are said to be removed if they are applied with the following fig wart tincture as strongly as possible 1-2 times a day.

## FIG WART TINCTURE

- 20 ml echinacea tincture

> - 20 ml arborvitae tincture
> - 20 ml marigold tincture
> - 10 ml celandine juice
>
> Mix all ingredients well. The mixture lasts a maximum of 3 weeks if kept cold.

## 134.  DROPSY, EDEMA

Edema was very common and a big problem in earlier times.

Mostly diuretics were used, which were supposed to promote the drainage of excess water.

Elderberry jam made from ripe elderberries was considered a good remedy for dropsy.

The elder root was a very old remedy for dropsy and was used as a decoction or as juice pressed from the inner bark.

Juniper berries were used as tea or as brandy, as well as horseradish root, which was taken as juice or mixed with beer.

The root of the spiny restharrow (Ononis spinosa) was used as tea. Sometimes it was also used together with wormwood and bogbean (Menyanthes trifoliata).

Garlic was also used. It was eaten raw or the juice was taken in broth.

Field horsetail, as well as carrot seeds, swamp reed grass (Calamagrostis canescens), were used as tea.

The root of the celandine was mixed with beer and drunk against dropsy, especially in Poland.

The roots of the German iris (Iris germanica) were pressed and a tablespoon was taken. This was supposed to cause watery diarrhea.

A decoction of black horehound (Ballota nigra) was also used.

Raw, unripe pineapple is said to be strongly diuretic.

As diuretic foods, parsley, celery, watercress, and asparagus were used.

## 135.     AGUE, MALARIA

The formerly common ague, also known as marsh fever, was a type of malaria transmitted particularly in the humid marshes of Northern Germany by the mosquito Anopheles atroparvus. This disease had been eradicated for many years. However, due to the desire to restore as much nature as possible to its original state, large areas that were previously drained are now being re-wetted. As a result, mosquitoes of the species Anopheles atroparvus can again be found in these areas, which could potentially lead to a resurgence of ague.

In some regions, a lot of physical activity and a daily glass of Madeira wine were considered good remedies.

Cold immersion baths followed by vigorous rubbing with towels were also deemed helpful. Saunas and sweating in steam baths were regionally common practices.

Additionally, compresses made from mustard flour and vinegar or crushed garlic were believed to be effective. The biting stonecrop (Sedum acre) was also used as a compress against ague and malaria. Sometimes it was mixed with salt and vinegar. Other remedies used in compresses included ginger, buttercup (Ranunculus acris), pepper, houseleek (Sempervivum tectorum), celandine, elder leaves, herb Robert (Geranium robertianum), marsh marigold (Caltha palustris) flowers, sage, field pennycress (Thlaspi arvense), rue (Ruta graveolens), among others.

Some people also used slices of white water lily (Nymphaea alba) tied to the soles of the feet.

Among old sailors, grog, coffee with rum, strong wine, brandy, juniper brandy, and punch were the preferred remedies.

Other plants believed to be helpful included birch bark steeped in brandy, bitter clover and wormwood as tinctures, as well as bird cherry (Prunus padus) bark, dandelion roots, calamus, olive leaves, boneset (Eupatorum perfoliatum) herb, 1-3 autumn crocus (Colchicum autumnale) flowers, pepperweed (Lepidium ruderale), pomegranate peel, usually boiled as tea, chewed, or used as a tincture.

Paste made from Madonna lily bulbs, applied as a compress, was also believed to be helpful.

The root bark of tulip tree (Liliodendron tulipifera), as well as the bark of smoke tree (Cotinus coggygria) or the leaves of European holly (Ilex aquifolium), were considered remedies against malaria. They were mostly brewed as tea.

Although cinchona bark was certainly a better remedy, it was sometimes unavailable due to trade restrictions and its very high price.


## 136.　　MENOPAUSE, HOT FLASHES

Flaxseeds are also believed to be helpful when chewed or incorporated into foods. A decoction of flaxseeds was also prepared and consumed.

### FLAXSEED DECOCTION

> 2 tbsp flaxseeds were soaked overnight in 2 cups of cold water and left covered. In the morning, the liquid was consumed, and the seeds were eaten.

Evening primrose, taken as tea or oil, is said to promote inner calmness and prevent hot flashes.

Drinking tea made from yarrow, red clover, sage, or dried juniper berries is believed to alleviate menopausal symptoms. These teas were consumed up to 3 times a day, one cup each.

### RED CLOVER TEA

> 1-2 tsp red clover steeped in 1 cup of boiling water, let it infuse for 5 minutes, then strain.

## JUNIPER BERRY TEA

> 1 tsp juniper berries steeped in 1 cup of boiling water, let it infuse for 10 minutes, then strain.

Nettle tea was also a proven home remedy for hot flashes during menopause.

Enjoying plenty of vegetables and dairy products while avoiding meat, chocolate, coffee, and sugar minimizes symptoms.

Engaging in regular exercise, preferably outdoors, helps prevent and alleviate symptoms.

Mistletoe tea was consumed for menopausal symptoms.

## 137.  WHITE DISCHARGE, VAGINAL DISCHARGE

Most often, sitz baths with additives such as chamomile, horsetail, or meadowsweet were the first choice.

Herbal tea was also used.

- 5 tbsp Walnut leaves
- 3 tbsp Purple loosestrife
- 3 tbsp Myrtle leaves
- 2 tbsp Shepherd's purse
- 2 tbsp Chamomile

Mix everything well. Steep 1 tsp of this mixture with boiling water, cover and let it infuse for 10 minutes, then strain and drink slowly. Drink one cup in the morning, one at noon, and one in the evening.

## 138.    TOOTHACHE

For toothaches, it was recommended to chew on a clove.

But also, a piece of root from the herb called Bertram, which was also known as tooth root in earlier times, was chewed. If the teeth had cavities, a piece of Bertram was inserted or a Bertram root decoction was prepared. For this, the root was boiled with wine or vinegar and used to rinse and gargle the mouth.

Rinsing, gargling, or drinking chamomile tea was also recommended.

Some also inserted a piece of wedge-shaped cut root of Plantain into the ear.

A remedy for toothaches was also rinsing with vinegar-larch needle decoction, vinegar-boiled elderberry root, or the decoction of Ground-ivy boiled in water.

In Russia, it was common to gargle with or rinse the mouth with the decoction of nettles boiled in wine vinegar.

## VINEGAR-LARCH NEEDLE DECOCTION

Boil 3 tbsp of fresh, crushed larch needles in a cup of wine vinegar and let the decoction steep for another 10 minutes covered. This decoction is used for rinsing the mouth and gargling.

## 139.          WORMS

Worms were a significant problem in early times. Even small children were often afflicted with roundworms. Hence, one finds in ancient literature numerous remedies against worm infestation. Below is a small excerpt of corresponding tips.

One of the most effective remedies against worms is to eat milk and garlic.

Also, eating a few chopped garlic cloves in the morning is said to expel worms, as well as herring salad with plenty of onions and garlic.

Drinking vinegar is also said to make the worms flee.

Other tips include eating raw carrots, drinking boiled carrot juice or honey. Especially for children, taking 1 tbsp of honey in the morning was recommended.

But also, cooking stinging nettle seeds in milk, rosehip seeds in honey, elderberry jam, tansy seeds with honey on bread, peppermint tea, acorn coffee, honey cake with worm seeds (seeds from Jerusalem oak - Dysphania anthelmintica), sauerkraut brine, ribwort plantain seeds, lemon seeds cooked in milk, 1 g powdered mayapple herb (Podophyllum peltatum) were the preferred methods to expel worms.

For roundworms, large amounts of asparagus were eaten, or birch sap was drunk.

For pinworms, which often afflict children and cause unbearable itching around the anus, grated raw carrots were given.

Inserting a piece of bacon attached to a string into the anus of infected children and pulling it out after some time is said to attract a large number of pinworms onto it, providing relief for a while.

Enemas with various additives such as milk, wormwood, valerian, tansy, orange peel, olive oil, lime water, and many others were administered.

For tapeworms, drinking plenty of cold water or mineral water was recommended.

Even Democritus recommended drinking a boiled infusion of peppermint against tapeworms.

In Iceland, it was customary to take ground charcoal against tapeworms.

Also, eating large quantities of wild strawberries or consuming them in the evening with sugar and wine was believed to expel tapeworms.

Raspberries and cherries, beans and sauerkraut, herring salad or anchovy salad with plenty of onions and garlic were believed to be particularly helpful.

Eating pickled olives and drinking almond oil was also thought to drive away tapeworms. This should be repeated every 30 minutes until the worm departs. Sometimes up to 1 kg of olives may be necessary.

## 140.     MUMPS

For mumps, bed rest was also recommended.

Sometimes, the neck was kept warm with a scarf or hot water bottle, and occasionally, compresses with cold quark were applied.

If the hands and feet were warm and the children had high fever, cooling calf wraps were administered.

As for food, a light diet was typically provided, often consisting of porridges and soups.

Chicken soup, in particular, was commonly used.